"Dr. Kathryn Schmitz is one of the world's leading researchers and advocates for the benefits of exercise for cancer patients. In her must-read book, Dr. Schmitz outlines the importance of beginning evidence-based, prescribed exercise programs before treatments commence, as well as through all stages of treatment and post-treatment. Her program will hopefully become a guiding light for all cancer patients."

—JAY K. HARNESS, MD, FACS

"In *Moving Through Cancer,* world-renowned expert Dr. Kathryn Schmitz shares what she has learned from her many research studies, her experience leading the American College of Sports Medicine, and her advocacy for exercise and cancer. This book is a must-read for cancer patients and survivors, their caregivers, and clinicians providing exercise advice and support."

—ANNE MCTIERNAN, MD, PhD, Fred Hutchinson Cancer Research **Center,** and author of *Cured: A Doctor's Journey from Panic to Peace*

"Every cancer patient and caregiver needs to read this book. If you're affected by cancer, it will inspire you to get moving, show you what you need to do (even on your darkest days) and hold your hand every step of the way. If you treat cancer patients, it will remind you why exercise should be the first treatment you recommend."

—DR. LIZ O'RIORDAN, coauthor of *The Complete Guide to Breast Cancer*

"A practical, scientifically based, heartfelt book to help patients successfully move through cancer. A must read for both patients and caregivers!"

—SUSAN GILCHRIST, MD, MD Anderson Cancer Center

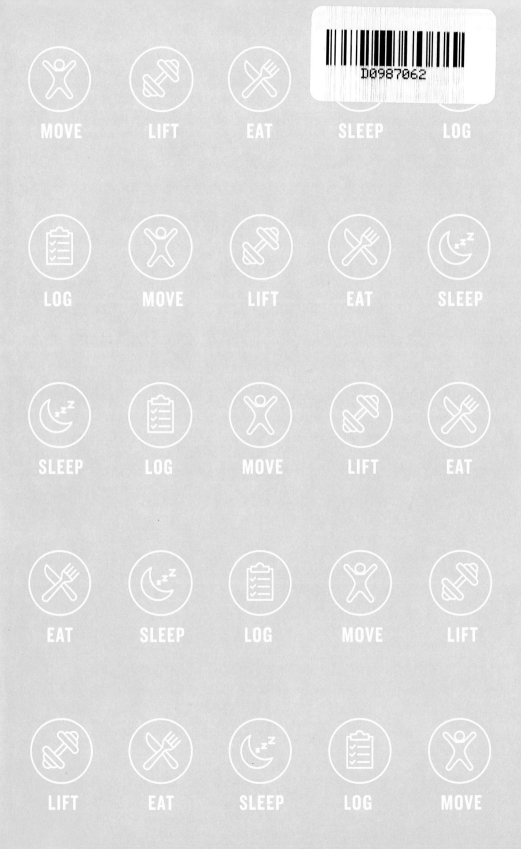

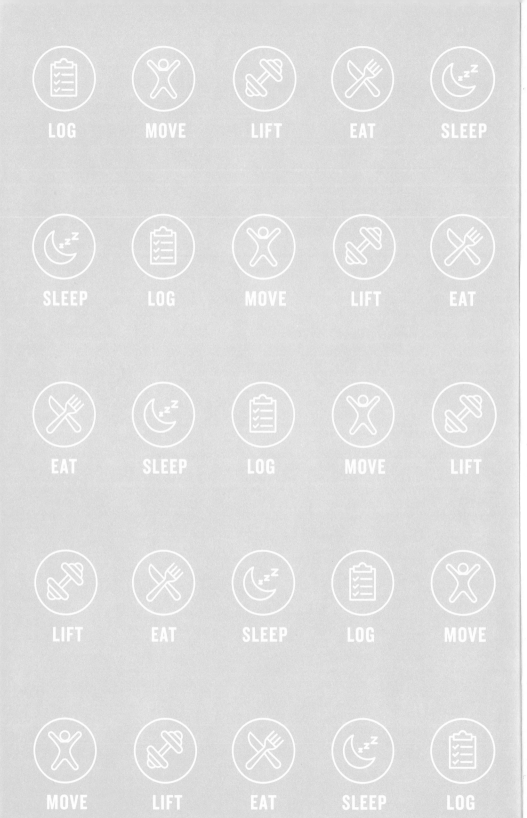

Advance Praise for MOVING THROUGH CANCER

"I have personally felt the helplessness of having cancer. Exercise was something I could control to help me face treatment and recover. This book beautifully translates a large body of research on exercise for cancer patients and gives them a practical approach to get started and stick with it! I highly recommend this book for any cancer patient and for oncology health care providers."

—NATALIE MARSHALL, MD, Medical Director, UCSF—John Muir
Health Cancer Center in Berkeley, and cancer survivor

"Finally, a book that celebrates and proves the importance of 'moving through cancer'! I love how this book breaks down the science of why it's so important to keep moving through treatment, highlighting the benefits for the body and the mind. I found the real stories of athletes who kept exercising through their treatment so relatable and inspiring. The book left me feeling hopeful and armed with confidence in the power of movement! This is a must read for anyone facing cancer!"

—KIKKAN RANDALL, US Olympic gold medalist in cross-country
skiing and cancer survivor

"After twenty-six years researching the benefits of exercise for cancer patients, Dr. Kathryn Schmitz and her wife, Sara, experience firsthand the restorative power of exercise as a part of cancer treatment. Providing both inspiration and guidance to patients facing their own cancer journeys, this personal narrative helps answer the all-too-common question asked by cancer patients: 'Doctor, what can I do myself to help me feel better?'"

—JENNIFER LIGIBEL, MD, Dana Farber Cancer Institute and Harvard
Medical School

MOVING THROUGH CANCER

MOVING THROUGH

CANCER

AN EXERCISE AND STRENGTH-TRAINING
PROGRAM FOR THE FIGHT OF YOUR LIFE

DR. KATHRYN SCHMITZ

WITH GABRIEL MILLER

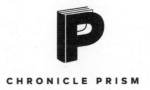

CHRONICLE PRISM

Figure in chapter 4 reprinted with permission from: William L. Haskell. "Health consequences of physical activity: understanding and challenges regarding dose-response." *Med. Sci. Sports Exerc* 26, no. 6 (1994): 649–660, 1994. https://journals.lww.com/acsm-msse/Abstract/1994/06000/Health_consequences_of_physical_activity_.1.aspx. Figure in chapter 7 reprinted with permission from: Amy A. Kirkham, Kelcey A. Bland, David S Zucker, Joshua Bovard, Tamara Shenkier, Donald C. McKenzie, Margot K. Davis, Karen A. Gelmon, Kristin L. Campbell. "Chemotherapy-periodized' exercise to accommodate for cyclical variation in fatigue." *Med. Sci. Sports Exerc* 52, no. 2 (2020): 278–86. https://journals.lww.com/acsm-msse/Fulltext/2020/02000/_Chemotherapy_periodized__Exercise_to_Accommodate.2.aspx.

Medicine and Science in Sports and Exercise is the flagship journal of the American College of Sports Medicine. The American College of Sports Medicine advances and integrates scientific research to provide educational and practical applications of exercise science and sports medicine. www.acsm.org.

Figure in chapter 5 reprinted with permission from: Francesco Carli, Chelsia Gillis, Celena Scheede-Bergdahl. "Promoting a culture of prehabilitation for the surgical cancer patient." *Acta Oncologica* 56, no. 2 (2017): 128–133, 2017. Reprinted by permission of the publisher: Taylor and Francis Ltd, http://www.tandfonline.com.

Moving Through Cancer is also the name of an initiative of the American College of Sports Medicine. https://www.exerciseismedicine.org/support_page.php/moving-through-cancer/.

Library of Congress Cataloging-in-Publication Data is available.

ISBN 978-1-7972-1025-4

Manufactured in the United States of America.

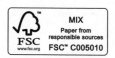

MIX
Paper from responsible sources
FSC www.fsc.org   FSC™ C005010

Design by Pamela Geismar.
Typesetting by Maureen Forys,
Happenstance Type-O-Rama. Typeset in
Adobe Garmond, Archer, and Knockout.

10 9 8 7 6 5 4 3 2 1

Chronicle books and gifts are available at special quantity discounts to corporations, professional associations, literacy programs, and other organizations. For details and discount information, please contact our premiums department at corporatesales@chroniclebooks.com or at 1-800-759-0190.

CHRONICLE PRISM

Chronicle Prism is an imprint of
Chronicle Books LLC
680 Second Street
San Francisco, California 94107

www.chronicleprism.com

To all the men and women living with and beyond cancer who have participated in exercise oncology trials. This book is possible because of you.

PART ONE

HOW
EXERCISE
HELPS

IT STARTS
WITH A PHONE CALL

t often starts with a phone call. A biopsy and weeks of waiting. Then the dreaded news: You. Have. Cancer.

What follows is a flurry of appointments and a plan for treatment. Time and again, you are told to rest, not to push yourself, because cancer treatment is tough enough as it is. Some patients recover from surgery, only to begin chemotherapy. Other patients endure endless months of chemotherapy without surgery. Is it possible to feel this tired? You then continue treatment, possibly with radiation or maintenance therapy. When it's all over, you ring that bell at the end of treatment feeling victorious.

And yet, you also feel like you have aged a decade over the past few months. A year later, you're still dealing with fatigue, neuropathy, and lymphedema. Does it have to be this way?

The answer is clear: No.

YOU CAN DO IT

As a leading clinical exercise oncology researcher for the past two decades, I had helped thousands of people with cancer in my research studies, but I did not really understand the process of living through a cancer diagnosis and treatment until my then-girlfriend and now-wife, Sara, was diagnosed with stage 3 cancer four years ago. It changed me forever and it changed the way that I have approached every patient since.

When you have that conversation that changes your life forever, a dark cloud comes over you. For perhaps the first time in your life, you realize, *I am mortal.* Or in my case, *My girlfriend is mortal.* For others, it's a spouse, a parent, or a close friend. You recognize that this disease can kill. That you're not going to live forever.

For Sara and me, this happened on an October morning in 2016, when we found out that she had stage 3 squamous cell carcinoma in her nose. A week later, we attended an appointment with surgical, radiation, and medical oncologists, as well as a nurse navigator and a social worker. Our first thought was that the room was too crowded for something so benign. About halfway through the meeting, Sara started to cry. The doctors were making it clear to both of us that this was not some "mild skin cancer" as we had mistakenly assumed—this was an aggressive, invasive cancer that would require significant surgery, likely radiation, and perhaps chemotherapy.

We kept thinking that someone had made a mistake, so we sought a second opinion. The answer was consistent: aggressive squamous cell carcinoma in the nasal passage that had spent the past year spreading across both nostrils and up through the skin.

We were told to come back in a month for surgery on Sara's nose. That's it. Nothing about what we might do in the intervening four weeks to give Sara the best chance of a good outcome. This is not uncommon, even though—as you have likely wondered and will learn about in this book—gaining whatever fitness you can *before* starting treatment is one of the best strategies to improve your chances of beating cancer.

In that moment with Sara, I was so freaked out, so completely blinded and overwhelmed by this life-changing diagnosis, that even as a clinical exercise oncology expert with 260 published scientific papers, I failed to see how exercise during this crucial window may have helped. In retrospect, I can see that she lost so much body weight, nearly all of which was muscle in her case. She lost so much ground. There was an opportunity there, and I could kick myself for not getting her a really good dose of strength training before she began the most difficult physical challenge of her life.

Sara was understandably angry at her diagnosis. Had it been caught six months earlier, it is very likely that her cancer would have been much easier to treat. Sara took incredible care of herself, going to her doctor regularly, eating well, exercising, and taking supplements to ward off disease. How could she, of all people, have an aggressive advanced cancer?

It is a very common experience to feel angry after a cancer diagnosis. You can feel like your body has let you down. This is true of everyone, but might be particularly true for people who are fit, have a normal weight, and eat a healthy diet. They feel like they've done everything right and yet *they still got cancer*. The only comfort I could give to Sara is that it could have been so much worse if she had been in bad shape, eating a bad diet, overweight, and smoking. Her cancer might have come on earlier and it might have been much more difficult to treat. But the process of developing cancer was going to happen regardless. Even if your lifestyle choices weren't perfect before your cancer, there is no value in blaming yourself. The cancer has happened. The only thing to do is to move forward.

It wasn't until later, when Sara was going through chemo and radiation and she started to have symptoms that I'm used to treating in my own research studies that I realized, *Oh wait, I can help.* I still remember the moment I recognized that she had lymphedema (swelling) in her face. My most well-known research study was about exercise and breast cancer–related lymphedema, published in the *New England Journal of Medicine* and *JAMA*. I knew all of the scientific evidence about how exercise and movement help cancer patients, and I knew that exercise was going to be particularly beneficial for Sara. She is petite, and maintaining muscle mass was going to be crucial (she didn't have much to begin with!). Further, to stave off loss of overall function and maintain her energy levels, aerobic exercise would be particularly helpful. I started making her walk on the treadmill in our home while she was going through combined chemotherapy and radiation. But even knowing what

I knew, I was conflicted. I saw how tired she was and how she desperately did not want to do it most days. I advised her to walk up to 30 minutes, but also to notice how the activity altered her fatigue and to back off if symptoms worsened. I am aware that some who read this book will wonder whether I am crazy to ask cancer patients to exercise as they are undergoing treatment. But YOU CAN DO IT, and I promise you, if you do, you're going to feel better.

I made Sara exercise, a least a little bit every day. Even though I felt so mean. But at the same time, I am absolutely convinced that Sara got through her full dosage of radiation and chemo on schedule because of it, with no need for breaks, no hospitalizations, and no reductions in dosage. In head and neck cancer, as well as some other cancers, chemo and radiation are given as a combined treatment at the same time. And it is just horrible. Thirty-five percent of head and neck cancer patients end up in the hospital during combined chemotherapy and radiation because of side effects that become too severe to manage at home. Yet Sara got through the whole thing with flying colors, and we are convinced that regular exercise helped. It can help you too. You CAN do it.

After she completed all of her surgeries, Sara began to feel stronger. And that is when we found boxing. That was when Sara really got her mojo back. It was clear to see that she was fighting back—literally. If my failure to recognize how exercise might help Sara before treatment was a low point, then this was a high one for us: seeing how exercise and boxing in particular empowered Sara to take back her life and feel strong again.

Being with Sara before and during her treatment and seeing every moment of her cancer journey has changed me in many ways. One is the way that I talk to patients with cancer about exercise. Prior to Sara's diagnosis, I would often simply think, *Well, of course exercise would be important, right?* But watching Sara go through it made it very personal. Sara's experience was somewhat different in that she had more surgeries than most cancer patients (five reconstructive surgeries over the course of two years). But it was quite typical in the sense that her cancer treatment was the hardest period of our lives. And it was very typical in the sense that she had incredibly empowering days in the boxing gym and then days where she was so tired from treatment that she couldn't drag herself off the couch if her life depended on it.

So my expectations have shifted. I recognize that the first thing I need to do when approaching someone with cancer to talk about their exercise is to simply be with that person, period. And if we can figure out what their particular challenges are and how we can address them through exercise, then we can really get to work.

IT'S SIMPLE AND ESSENTIAL: JUST GET UP AND MOVE

The idea that exercise benefits people living with cancer is nothing new. In 2005, researcher Michelle Holmes published the first of what has become a library of epidemiologic research documenting the benefits of being more active after a cancer diagnosis. Dr. Holmes, a Harvard epidemiologist, used data from the Nurses' Health Study to show that breast cancer survivors who were more active had a lower risk of breast cancer mortality. More specifically, women who walked 3 to 5 hours per week reduced their risk of breast cancer mortality by half. The following year, my colleague, Dr. Jeffrey Meyerhardt, a medical oncologist, also from Harvard, published similar findings for colorectal cancer survivors. Dr. Meyerhardt observed a reduction of cancer-specific mortality of over 60 percent for colorectal cancer survivors who did more than 18 MET-hours per week of physical activity (MET-hours is a unit of describing time and intensity of exercise. For example, 18 MET-hours is roughly equivalent to 5 to 6 hours a week of walking).

The field didn't start there: A study was published in 1938 with convincing data in animals that exercise slows the growth of cancerous tumors. We've had evidence on the effects of exercise on cancer for more than eighty years!

In the 1980s, nursing scientists Maryl Winningham and Mary MacVicar carried out the first randomized controlled exercise trials in cancer patients, the first of which was published in 1988. They observed positive effects of cycling exercise on aerobic fitness, symptoms, and body composition in their breast cancer research participants. In 1996, two well-known Canadian scientists, Christine Friedenreich and Kerry Courneya, surveyed the best research studies that had been completed of exercise in cancer patients. They found four pilot studies, including the work of Winningham and MacVicar. In 2005, I collected all of the published clinical trials on exercise in cancer patients and compared their results. At the time, I found twenty-two clinical trials. Five years later, I did the exact same search and found nearly three times as many. Sensing that we were at the beginning of a groundswell, I led the publication that provided the first exercise and cancer recommendations from the American College of Sports Medicine. This was followed shortly by similar recommendations from two leading cancer groups, the American Cancer Society and the National Comprehensive Cancer Network. One of the major goals of all of these recommendations was to put oncology doctors and nurses on notice that the days of telling cancer patients to "rest, take it easy, don't push yourself" were over. The first two words of our recommendations in 2010 (and again in 2019) were AVOID INACTIVITY.

After the publication of the first American College of Sports Medicine roundtable guidelines, the field really exploded. Between 2010 and 2019, the number of published research papers on exercise and cancer went from fewer than a hundred to more than a thousand. We had reached a tipping point. It was clear that the scientific community understood just how important movement and exercise are for people fighting cancer. That year I organized a much larger group of researchers—representatives from seventeen cancer and exercise organizations around the world, including the American Cancer Society and the National Cancer Institute—to come together and update our recommendations on how much and what kinds of exercise people with cancer should try to do.

For this, we looked at all of the major published research on the subject—and the findings were conclusive. The publications from Holmes and Meyerhardt were the first, but dozens of observational epidemiologic studies now support a strong role for exercise in preventing cancer-specific and overall mortality, particularly in breast, colorectal, and prostate cancer survivors. And exercise is especially effective in reducing the risk of developing some of the most common cancers, including colon, breast, endometrial, kidney, bladder, esophageal, and stomach cancers.

But very importantly, the benefits don't end there. Exercise *after you have been diagnosed* actually changes the trajectory of your cancer. In studies in animals, for example, exercise changes the molecular environment around some tumors, slowing or even stopping their growth. And most importantly, in several major studies in people, exercise reduces their likelihood of dying from cancer and increases their chance of living longer.

One of these studies took 242 women who were about to start chemotherapy and divided them into three groups. One group would do aerobic exercise during treatment, including activities like biking, jogging, and walking. Another would do strength training instead. The final group wouldn't change anything during their treatment.

These researchers then waited and watched the women in the study for eight years to see whether exercising during their treatment had any effect. Specifically, they were looking at how long each of the women went without any signs or symptoms of cancer, which is a common way of measuring how well a treatment for cancer works.

When they compared who fared better, those who exercised were 7 percent more likely to be cancer free. Put another way, for every fourteen people who did a simple exercise routine during their cancer, one of them was cancer free because of it.

This same group of Canadian researchers then looked at whether continuing to exercise throughout treatment or starting a program and then quitting had any effect in a group of people with lymphoma. This is important for a couple of reasons. One is that a study like this can help point out whether more exercise is better than less. Another is that, as we'll discuss much more in this book, exercising during cancer is often hard—a lot of different factors can get in the way. A study like this can point out the importance of trying to stick with regular exercise.

Not surprisingly, those who did not exercise at all fared worse than those who did. But interestingly, there weren't any major differences in people who exercised regularly but missed a few days here and there and those who almost never missed an exercise session. And very importantly, there was another group that fared very well: those who began their treatment without doing any exercise at all, but then decided halfway through to start exercising.

Another study focused on more than 330 women who had just undergone surgery for breast cancer. One group did a simple exercise program for eight months after they had recovered from surgery; the other did not. Eight years after surgery, this simple exercise program had reduced these women's risk of dying by half.

These three studies are important because they divided up the people into groups *before* their cancer treatment. In addition to this type of clinical trial research, twenty-three more of the most rigorous, high-quality epidemiologic observational research studies assessing how exercise affects the survival of cancer patients—done in people with breast, prostate, and colon cancer—show very convincingly that regular exercise done *after* you've been diagnosed with cancer can reduce your chances of dying from this disease by as much as 69 percent.

When we released the results of the American College of Sports Medicine's Roundtable on Exercise for Cancer Prevention and Control in 2019, it was news around the world. At the time, the *New York Times* published our simple advice, which I will discuss in detail in this book: "Get up. Move. It's so simple and so essential. Get up and move."

One of the major goals of the recently published guidelines by the American College of Sports Medicine was to help make exercise the standard of care for all people living with and beyond cancer. We were pained to read in the scientific literature that only 9 percent of nurses and around 20 percent of physicians who treat cancer talk to their patients about exercise. The reasons are myriad, often focused on the limited time available during medical appointments and a belief that patients would not be receptive. However, the results of a major survey undertaken by the American Society of Clinical Oncology were encouraging—they revealed that the vast majority of medical oncologists agree that their patients would benefit from exercise during and after cancer treatment. And we know already that people with cancer are interested in exercising. In one 2019 survey, 95 percent of cancer patients said they felt that regular activity and exercise were very important during their cancer treatment, and the majority of them recognized the benefits: overall well-being, maintaining function, and reducing stress.

One benefit of the explosion in research on exercise and cancer is that we can look at more and more specific questions in our studies, such as what "dose" of exercise should be recommended for a specific problem or to try and achieve a specific outcome. This is the other major step forward that we have only just recently been able to take: We can now "dose" exercise for specific cancer-related problems in exactly the same way that your oncologist might prescribe a drug or chemotherapy regimen.

Ten years ago, all we could say was "Yes, you should exercise. We believe it is better for you. And there are a few reasons why we think this works, but we can't really tell you exactly how much, how often, or what intensity would work best, even though we think it might work this way." A decade later, we can actually prescribe exercise for eight different, very specific problems that people with cancer care about—anxiety, depression, fatigue, quality of life, lymphedema, physical function, bone health, and sleep. We now have specific exercises and exercise programs that anyone can do—exercises that I will describe in depth throughout this book—that reduce anxiety and depression, improve fatigue and physical function, and lead to better sleep and bone health. We also know that exercise does not increase the risk of developing lymphedema, a very common and debilitating side effect of cancer treatments.

We can also now say, for example, that if you have breast cancer, aerobic exercise like vigorous walking or light cycling for just 30 minutes three times a week will improve the debilitating fatigue that often accompanies cancer treatment—you don't need any more to see a benefit. But if you want to, you can certainly do this exercise five days a week or add some strength training, which will continue to incrementally improve your symptoms.

We can say with certainty that exercise before, during, and after cancer treatment improves many side effects of surgery, radiation, and cancer drugs; improves your chances of making it through treatment without needing to take a break; and improves your chances of living longer after your treatments are finished.

CHERYL'S STORY

My former research participant Cheryl Hogle's story is representative of how exercise during and after cancer treatment can not only change your body but your mindset as well. Her experience also illustrates how some longstanding—and incorrect—assumptions about exercise during cancer have prevented it from helping more people.

Now a recently retired teacher's aide in Edina, Minnesota, Cheryl was diligent about getting regular mammograms and cancer screenings. So when she noticed some redness on one side of her breast that didn't seem to go away, she went to her doctor. Thinking it was an infection, he prescribed her a course of antibiotics. He also referred her to a breast surgeon. The appointment with the breast surgeon was a week later, after she had finished the first course of antibiotics. The redness had not gone away, so the breast surgeon prescribed a second course of anti-biotics. When the redness didn't go away, Cheryl asked her primary care doctor for a referral to a new surgeon who requested that she undergo an ultrasound, which turned up negative, followed by a biopsy. He told her he didn't think she had cancer but that he wanted to be sure.

In fact, the biopsy came back positive for cancer. As is common, Cheryl's first cancer treatment was surgery, and when the surgeons went into her breast to remove the cancerous tissue, it was found in her lymph nodes as well. Within three weeks, Cheryl had had three surgeries and was suddenly looking at a 50-50 chance of surviving to five years. Her treatment included chemotherapy and radiation, as well as five years of tamoxifen, an estrogen blocker, to keep the cancer from returning.

Her lymphedema showed up almost exactly one year after her diagnosis. Lymphedema is swelling in any part of the body that happens when excess fluid gets backed up in the lymphatic system. It is very common in the arms and torso after breast cancer surgery and can be very uncomfortable and achy, as well as limit movement.

I met Cheryl when a mutual friend, a massage therapist, mentioned that she might be a good candidate for a research study that I was working on to test whether it was safe for women with lymphedema after breast cancer surgery to lift weights. At the time, Cheryl told me that she never exercised. In fact, she said she had never been in a gym before.

In this study, we showed these women the strength exercises that we wanted them to do (including all those included in chapters 5 through 11 of this book) and gave them a packet with pictures and step-by-step instructions. We supervised them in the gym for thirteen weeks. Then we asked them to do the same program of weight-lifting exercises on their own for another thirteen weeks.

When Cheryl first walked into the gym, she had lost so much strength and function in her arm that she had trouble opening a water bottle. The lymphedema had made her arm so puffy and tight that she could not reach for things over her head. Everyday things like carrying groceries had become difficult, sometimes insurmountable, tasks.

A regular program of resistance training, starting with very low weights, gave Cheryl her strength and flexibility back by the end of the first half of the program. But more importantly, it empowered her during a time when so much felt out of her control.

"When you get a serious cancer diagnosis, it really throws you," Cheryl said. "Exercising gave me a way of being proactive. There is a psychological impact of getting lymphedema that is not only physical. We started at pretty low weights and I was able to make good progression through the study. That was very empowering. Because you do really want that part of your life back—when you feel like you can do the things that you want to do. Swim, play tennis, gardening—whatever activity it is you did before."

Cheryl felt so empowered, in fact, that she started a support group for women like herself with lymphedema after breast surgery. "Doing the whole exercise program encouraged me to step out and do this," Cheryl said. "This is not something I would have said before, 'Oh, let's be the Twin Cities Lymphedema Support Group.'"

The idea behind the group was to gather the collective knowledge of women in Minneapolis and Saint Paul living with lymphedema as a chronic condition so that they could support each other and those newly diagnosed with it. It was needed, they felt, because many of the women had oncologists or breast surgeons who didn't really know much about treating or managing lymphedema.

"I had great physicians. But I think they were just so focused on the treatment. You go to a surgeon and all they want to think about is surgery," Cheryl said. "I remember going back to my surgeon for a checkup and saying, 'You know, I can't raise my arm that well.' And he said, 'Well, sometimes that happens.' And I'm like, 'OK, that's not really a good solution.'"

This is a typical experience for people with cancer. It's the same with exercise. During Cheryl's treatment, none of her doctors mentioned exercise, nor have they during her more than ten years as a survivor.

It isn't that doctors don't recognize the benefits of regular exercise for people living with cancer. In fact, the opposite is true: Cancer doctors overwhelmingly wish their patients exercised. One recent study of more than 900 cancer doctors, nurses, and physician assistants found that 80 percent agreed they should be recommending physical activity to their patients.

And yet, as alluded to earlier, fewer than half of cancer doctors regularly mention exercise or physical activity to their patients, and fewer than a quarter actually refer their patients to an exercise program. The main reason, they say, is that they feel they lack the time to discuss exercise during already busy appointments, or they feel their patients would not be receptive to advice on exercise.

The truth, however, is that when faced with a life-changing cancer diagnosis, the overwhelming majority of cancer patients—as many as 90 percent—want their doctor to tell them how lifestyle choices like physical activity can improve their chances of beating their cancer.

So people with cancer want information about how exercise can help them. And their doctors want them to have it, even though they're not giving it to patients for a variety of reasons. That is why I'm writing this book: so that every cancer patient has this information and can benefit from all the ways that exercise helps during and after cancer treatment. In these pages I'm going to give you the same exercise programs that have helped Cheryl Hogle—and countless others—get their lives back and empowered them to beat cancer. The exercises I will describe fall into two categories: aerobic and strength training. *Aerobic exercise* refers to activities like brisk walking, swimming, running, or cycling. You probably know it as "cardio." Generally speaking, it's the kind of activity that increases your breathing and heart rate.

Strength training or *resistance training* is exercise that improves muscular strength and endurance. During these workouts, you push or pull your limbs against some form of resistance such as your own body weight, elastic bands, free weights (like dumbbells), or weight machines. Both exercise modalities have been shown to benefit people living with and beyond cancer and are important to the benefits described in this book. Let's get started!

NOW WHAT?

My wife, Sara, received the results of her biopsy on a Tuesday. For the rest of the week, she was in a daze. Then on Saturday it hit her, in the shower of all places, where she broke down sobbing for what felt like an eternity. We still had no idea what was going on, but for the first time it dawned on her just how vulnerable she was.

The next month was a whirlwind of appointments. "It's so hard to describe how I felt during that time because everything just moved so fast," she said. "I didn't have time to even think—I felt like I was on a treadmill and I had to cast my emotions aside."

We were told that Sara's treatment would consist of surgery to remove the tip of her nose as well as radiation to make sure that all of the cancer cells were killed. At first, it seemed promising—*just the tip of her nose and a bit of radiation!*—but as the surgery neared we began to get worried. It turned out the "tip" was her whole nose.

That was the first of many devastating realizations for us. By her own admission, Sara is a quiet, shy, and introverted person. She has said that, in her own way, she would prefer to go through life unnoticed, feeling no need to draw attention to herself.

With the diagnosis and the planned surgery, that was now shattered. "Someone told me that they were going to cut my entire nose off and that

I would be walking around with a hole in my face until reconstruction," Sara said. "People don't just 'lose their noses.' I felt like I was going to look like an absolute freak." She was worried about what I would think, what her family would think, what people in line at the coffee shop would think. "There were so many emotions that I can't even describe how many I had at that point," she said.

To add to the confusion, the reconstructive surgeon Sara met with advised that she undergo a reconstructive surgery known as a forehead flap, in which the skin on her forehead would be used to recreate her nose. He suggested doing the reconstruction six months after completing chemotherapy and radiation. We also sought the opinion of a second surgeon, who would do the reconstruction at the same time as the "complete rhinectomy" (complete removal of the nose). We chose to work with the second surgeon. "It made me feel so hopeful," she said. "I remember just basically going, 'Oh my God, I'm going to have a nose. It's as good as what I had before. This isn't going to be so bad.'"

All we felt we had to do was get through the curative treatment and the anticipated two additional reconstructive surgeries—about a year all told. But one of the cruel ironies of cancer is that despite all of the incredible imaging technologies available to doctors, they still do not know with certainty how serious your cancer is until you are under the knife. In the operating room, Sara's surgeon was faced with a terrible choice: because her cancer had traveled near her eye sockets, if he cut it all out she may have lost her vision. Instead, he decided to leave that little bit of cancer behind—along with her vision—and hope that it was killed during the chemotherapy and radiation after surgery.

During that following year, Sara had concurrent chemotherapy and radiation—treatments that knocked the very life right out of her and brought both of us to our knees emotionally. We also began the first of what would be five attempts by surgeons to reconstruct Sara's nose. After the last try, the surgeon finally said, "Sara, that's it. That's all we can do. The tissue can't handle any more." Sara never cried about her cancer the way that she cried after that. She went to her parents' house and cried for hours—she was crying so hard that she literally couldn't catch her breath.

Sara had kind, compassionate, skilled physicians treating her cancer and reconstructing her nose. They were wonderful people and incredible doctors. At the time, I was on the faculty at the University of Pennsylvania—these were my colleagues and they were world-class. But even given all of that, we were on an emotional roller coaster the entire time, by turns hopeful and completely devastated.

This is the nature of cancer. It is filled with uncertainty. It is a blur of anxiety and confusion. It is a total loss of control over your body. It's being forced to make decisions without feeling like you understand them. It's realizing that you don't even know the questions you should be asking. And even the very best doctors in the world do not know what your journey as a cancer patient is going to be.

There is no way to guarantee what your experience as a cancer patient will be, but I can guarantee that moving—getting some exercise, even just a little bit—will make you feel better. Study after study has shown that exercise leads to better quality of life, fitness, energy, and strength. And I can guarantee that if you don't, you will lose some physical part of your daily life—whether that's being able to open a pickle jar or run 10 miles—because of treatment. As you read this, you may be questioning whether you can exercise as you go through treatment. I do hear about this questioning from some patients. My promise to you is this: Try the exercises recommended in this book for 10 minutes. If you don't feel better, you can stop. But my deep experience tells me you will feel better.

When I worked with other experts at the American College of Sports Medicine to gather all of the scientific studies looking at how exercise affects people beyond their cancer itself—that is, how exercise changes their emotional and psychological well-being—we found the strongest evidence was for reducing anxiety and fighting depression, which so often follow the news that you have cancer.

Sara's journey was full of unexpected turns. But even when everything goes as planned, a cancer diagnosis is still incredibly confusing and difficult. In this moment, when everything is taken away from you, exercise is a powerful reminder that you do have control over your body and this experience of having cancer. And you can feel strong and powerful even when facing a difficult health crisis. As I've said before: You CAN do it.

As mentioned in the previous chapter, studies have shown that exercise during cancer treatment may actually improve your chances of living longer. One of the ways it might do this is by helping you get through all of your planned treatments on schedule, at the dose originally intended. This has strong implications for your long-term survival. Cancer treatments are draining, debilitating experiences, in part because they often involve delivering the largest dose your body can handle to maximize the treatment's effect. But sometimes, side effects become overwhelming, and you're forced to either lower your dose or stop it entirely while your body recovers, prolonging or reducing the total treatment dose received. Doing aerobic exercises like walking or riding a bicycle and strength training with weights or other types of resistance have been shown to increase a patient's chances of finishing treatment on time and with the originally planned dose.

Another way exercise may help is by spreading cancer drugs throughout your body more effectively. Researchers at the Centre for Physical Activity Research in Copenhagen have looked closely at this by comparing the way drugs move through the bodies of cancer patients who have exercised regularly and those who have not. They have found that chemotherapy drugs are distributed more widely in those who are physically fit, meaning that they are less likely to experience the kind of side effects that cause someone to reduce or stop their treatment. They also believe this happens when people start exercising immediately before or during chemotherapy treatments—the movement increases the flow of blood to the muscles, likely reducing the side effects of the drugs.

Exercise may also help patients complete their treatments by stimulating the body's natural defenses—the immune system. When you exercise, your body responds by increasing the number of immune cells circulating in your blood. This in turn may stimulate the bone marrow to produce new immune cells that further support the body's defense mechanisms. The loss of immune cells during cancer treatment is a very common reason for cancer patients to have to slow down or stop their treatments altogether.

These are just a few of the ways that exercise can help your body during cancer treatment. Let's take a look at how you can expect cancer and its treatment to affect your entire body. They can affect your body *locally*, such as the way surgery or focused radiation might change only one part of your body, or *systemically*, as in the way chemotherapy has the potential to do damage throughout your entire body. We'll also look at how exercise counteracts each one of these side effects.

Table 1. How Exercise Helps Your Body During Cancer Treatment

ORGAN/AREA OF THE BODY	EFFECT OF CANCER AND TREATMENT	HOW EXERCISE HELPS
Head	Cognitive changes	May protect against changes in cognitive function
	Anxiety	Reduces anxiety
	Depression	Protects against depression
	Sleep	Improves sleep quality
Chest	Cardiovascular system	May prevent or improve cardio-toxic effects of treatment by improving cardiac function
Arms	Lymphedema	Improves lymphedema symptoms in breast cancer
Hands/Feet	Peripheral neuropathy	Can improve mobility and balance
Reproductive	Decrease in sexual function	May help maintain or improve sexual function
Legs	Worsening bone health	Improves bone health
	Pain	May improve joint pain
	Fatigue	Reduces fatigue both during and after treatment
General	Immune system	Supports body's immune defenses
	Weight gain	Prevents weight gain
	Loss of muscle/strength	Helps maintain muscle mass and strength

WHAT TO EXPECT

While every person's journey with cancer is unique, Dr. Liz O'Riordan has a truly rare perspective: She was a breast cancer surgeon in the United Kingdom when, at the age of forty, she was diagnosed with stage 3 breast cancer herself. She'd spent her entire professional life learning about breast cancer and talking with women about their treatment and the likely course their breast cancer would take. And yet nothing in those years of training and experience prepared her for what it actually felt like to face her own cancer.

Like most patients, she was convinced the lump in her breast was another cyst. "After all, I should know what a cancer feels like, shouldn't I?" This turned out to be the first of many misconceptions she had as a breast cancer surgeon. "I used to tell women with small cancers that they were lucky we caught it early," she said. "No one is lucky to have cancer. The words you use as a doctor take on a different meaning when you're hearing them for the first time as a patient."

Like most time-strapped cancer doctors, when Dr. O'Riordan first delivered a cancer diagnosis to one of her patients, she also had to provide them with an enormous amount of other information: what treatment they need, whether they might need chemotherapy and radiotherapy, the complications of all those treatments, as well as dates for surgery, preoperative assessments, and follow-up appointments. However, when she was on the other side of this discussion—even knowing what to expect—she couldn't process any of it. "Instead of being able to focus on all the information I was being given, all I kept thinking was, '*Insert your own swear word*, I've got cancer.' When it was over and I had been given a plan, all I wanted to do was to run out of the room screaming."

Dr. O'Riordan's story is unique because she's a breast cancer surgeon. But her experience as a patient is very typical. Enormous numbers of cancer patients, even when being treated by compassionate, caring physicians, lack basic information about their treatment, including whether their condition is considered curable or not; if not, how long they can expect to live; or why they're being prescribed chemotherapy or radiation.

Much of this has to do with just how rushed the process is. "I felt like so much information was being thrown at me," Sara, my wife, told me. "It's so hard to even describe how I felt after my diagnosis because everything just moved so fast."

We liked and respected her oncologists. Yet we never felt fully prepared for anything that happened because everything felt like it was moving so quickly. "They're trying to tell you how they're going to basically change your life—inject chemicals into your body, remove your nose or your breast, for example, tell you about radiation, and they're doing all of this in like five to ten minutes," Sara said.

Researchers have spent a lot of time looking at how oncologists deliver news to cancer patients. In one study, they recorded 128 conversations between oncologists and their patients and then tracked how much time was spent discussing various aspects of the patient's experience: symptoms, treatments, logistics like scheduling appointments, or prognosis (how well or poorly a patient can expect to do). Regardless of the type of news being delivered—good, bad, or neutral—information about how the patient might expect to do in the future, their prognosis, was always less than 10 percent of the entire conversation. Symptoms and treatments dominated these conversations, and even discussions of upcoming appointments lasted longer than talking about how a cancer patient could expect to do during and after their treatment—in other words, how long they could expect to live and what their life would look like.

It isn't just the lack of time, or the complexity of cancer treatments, that make these discussions so confusing and difficult. Because cancer may be fatal, both oncologists and patients find discussing the negative aspects of treatment—including possibly death—very difficult. These are not easy conversations for anyone to have, so instead both doctors and patients often focus on hope and the next steps in treatment rather than talk about the sometimes brutal truth of a poor prognosis. No one wants to feel hopeless in the weeks after a cancer diagnosis, but this can leave cancer patients, like my wife, Sara, feeling like they never got the full picture of what to expect.

EXERCISE AS THE FOURTH TREATMENT FOR CANCER

When you are told you have cancer, your world is shattered. At the very least, you give up control of your body to surgery, chemo, or radiation—perhaps all three. You may be facing a lifelong side effect of cancer treatment, like nerve damage from chemotherapy or a colostomy bag after rectal cancer surgery. At worst, you have to face your own mortality much sooner than you ever expected.

When I spoke with Dr. O'Riordan about dealing with her own cancer diagnosis, she was unequivocal about how regular exercise helped her cope. "It was about cancer not defining me," she said. "I wasn't going to let cancer take everything away from me. It took my hair, it took my femininity, I lost my breast, I lost my ovaries, I lost my job, and I was off work sick. But I was like, 'It can't take exercise away from me.'" Dr. O'Riordan hadn't been an avid exerciser prior to her diagnosis. In fact, she had avoided sports for most of her life. It was the threat of losing the opportunity to exercise that motivated her to start.

"Just being outside in the fresh air exercising, I wasn't thinking about the fact that I had cancer. I was just enjoying being alive. And I also thought, 'I'm incredibly lucky to have two arms and two legs that work. And I want my body to be strong and fit enough to cope with whatever happens to it.'" This is true whether you have breast cancer like Dr. O'Riordan or any other type of cancer.

In one analysis that looked at the results of sixty-one clinical trials of women with breast cancer, those who exercised during treatment had better quality of life, fitness, energy, and strength, as well as significantly less anxiety and depression. A different analysis, this one including the experiences of more than 1,000 patients with a variety of advanced cancers, including leukemia; lymphoma; multiple myeloma; and lung, breast, gastrointestinal, and prostate cancers, found the exact same thing: Those who did regular exercise during cancer treatment had much better physical function, energy, psychological well-being, and overall quality of life.

Exercise is empowering. When your body is moving and working, more often than not your mind is free of worry and fear. You feel good because you know that you're taking care of yourself. You're alert, happy, and full of life.

"I think exercise should be the fourth treatment for cancer," said Dr. O'Riordan, who exercised all the way through chemotherapy, surgery, and radiotherapy, including completing half-Ironman triathlons and a 65-mile bike ride through the Alps. "It should be the fourth thing we prescribe. But with cancer, you've got everybody from a twenty-two-year-old elite runner to a seventy-year-old who can't stand up from a chair. There's not one prescription that fits all, and everybody's treatment is different and unique."

As you'll learn throughout this book, exercise can be prescribed exactly like other cancer treatments, with differing "doses" depending on your age, ability, and type of treatment. And, most importantly, the benefits of movement extend to everybody, whether you've never been to the gym a day in your life or you're a gold medal–winning Olympic athlete.

ONE THING IS CERTAIN: EXERCISE WILL HELP

Most likely, you or someone you know has experienced a cancer diagnosis. You're familiar, at least on some level, with just how difficult—often devastating—that news can be. And my hope is that by hearing the stories of my wife, Sara, breast cancer surgeon Liz O'Riordan, and others throughout the book, you take away one central message about this experience: Expect the unexpected. Your journey through cancer treatment will almost certainly not follow the path you expect it to. But one of the things we know for certain is that exercise is proven to help throughout this entire process, from before your very first treatment well into your years as a cancer survivor.

Importantly, the information that I've included in this book is based on sound science—a body of scientific evidence that we've been building for decades. And it continues to grow. In the next chapter, I'll tell you how to find your own scientifically accurate information as well as how to judge whether something you've found online is based on solid scientific evidence. I'll also talk about the kinds of scientific evidence and medical studies that I'm including in this book, so that you can rest assured that you're getting only the very best information as you move through cancer.

WHAT YOU WILL NEED

To follow the advice in this book, you will need tools. We describe them below, and you can download blank forms and examples from my website, www.movingthroughcancer.com.

A WAY TO TRACK YOUR AEROBIC EXERCISE

You will want to record your aerobic exercise daily (we'll get to that in a bit). Options include counting the minutes on a watch or stopwatch you already own. Alternatively, you may want to consider investing in a fitness tracker. Options range from a $20 pedometer to a smartwatch. Don't worry too much about the brand or version. For ideas and links, see my website, www.movingthroughcancer.com.

Having something that counts your steps or your time spent exercising is the goal. The value of having a tracker is twofold. First, it won't misremember how much you moved. We humans sometimes do. Second, there is published evidence that step counts can help predict whether someone will need to be hospitalized during combined chemotherapy and radiation treatments, as well as predict the ability to complete therapy, and even overall survival from cancer. As such, if your step counts start to decline, it might be worth sharing that with your cancer care team. It is an indication that you are feeling poorly and may need some kind of intervention to help with symptoms.

SOME KIND OF WEIGHTS

Throughout this book, we will ask you to do resistance training exercises. You will need weights of increasing heaviness to progress and continue improving your strength. This type of exercise is crucial to preventing the loss of muscle (and associated loss of function) that many people experience as a result of going through cancer treatment. I hear patients say all the time that they feel like they aged a decade during the months of cancer treatment. That feeling is the result of the loss of muscle and function. Resistance exercise before, during, and after treatment can help, and to do this, you will need some heavy things to lift. Options for this will include buying dumbbells a few pairs at a time. Generally weights cost $1 a pound. You could start by purchasing 3-, 5-, 8-, and 10-pound dumbbells (in pairs), which should cost around $50. You will likely need to eventually purchase 12-, 15-, and 20-pound dumbbells. Alternatively, you could purchase a set of adjustable dumbbells. Unlike the fitness tracker, the quality of adjustable dumbbells really can matter. For links to dumbbell sets and adjustable dumbbell kits that I've seen cancer patients use successfully, visit my website, www.movingthroughcancer.com.

A WAY TO RECORD YOUR SYMPTOMS AND WORKOUTS: THE LOG OR STAR CHART

Throughout the book, we will ask you to log your symptoms, reflect on your sleep, note your protein intake, and brag about your exercise. You will need a place to do that. Your caregiving team can help with this (see chapter 15 about caregiving). We've made a blank log (see page 26) you can use that includes the elements that will be referred to throughout this book. You can photocopy it directly out of the book or go to my website (www.movingthroughcancer.com) to download the page. Included in the log is the question of whether today is a "good" or a "bad" day. This will help you denote days with particularly difficult symptoms and might be most relevant directly after surgery or when you are undergoing chemotherapy or radiation treatments. The rest of the log is intended to help you keep track of how your symptoms and exercise behaviors are changing as you move through and beyond treatment. By keeping this log current, you will be able to help your doctors know when things are getting better or worse. This will help them know how you are responding to your treatments and when and how to provide medical support options. If you have a better idea, that's awesome. Share it with us on social media: @fitaftercancer on Twitter and @fitnessaftercancer on Instagram. Or share it in the community forum on my website, www.movingthroughcancer.com.

MOVING THROUGH CANCER LOG

	SUN	MON	TUE
GOOD DAY / BAD DAY			
FATIGUE 0 – 10 (10 = WORST)			
OTHER SYMPTOMS 0 – 10 (10 = WORST)			
SLEEP 0 – 10 (10 = BEST)			
MOVE* ★ (PER 30 MIN)			
LIFT ★ (PER SESSION)			
PROTEIN† # SERVINGS			

*The move goal varies according to where you are in treatment (less during chemotherapy and radiation). See chapters 5–11.

†See chapter 13 for guidance on how much protein you need. For the purposes of this chart, either add up the total grams of protein eaten each day or the number of servings: 1 serving = 3 oz of meat/poultry/fish, ½ cup cottage cheese or yogurt, 1 egg, 1 cup of milk, 1 cup of lentils/beans, or 1 protein drink/bar

WED	THU	FRI	SAT

NOTES:

_____
_____
_____
_____

THE SCIENTIFIC EVIDENCE

Historically, the prevailing assumption has been that cancer patients should rest, that they shouldn't overexert themselves because they need to save all of their energy to fight their cancer.

Ten years ago, when the American College of Sports Medicine (ACSM) first organized a group of experts on exercise and cancer to think about how we could convince more cancer doctors to recommend physical activity, our message reflected this reality. We knew we had to convince those who care for cancer patients that exercise was safe for their patients.

When ACSM convened a similar group a decade later, our message had completely flipped: Our first message, "exercise is not harmful during cancer treatment," had become "you're actually harming yourself by *not* exercising."

As I'll discuss later in this chapter, a lot of very important research came out during those intervening ten years. But other important changes happened as well. Newer drugs became available that were safer and had fewer, or less intense, side effects. Cancer treatment moved out of the hospital and into outpatient clinics, meaning that you arrived, received your treatment, and then left the same day. (Chemotherapy used to mean staying in the hospital for weeks at a time.) But perhaps most importantly, more and more cancer patients began carrying on with their lives despite being in the middle of cancer treatment. They felt well enough to work. They continued to be involved in their communities. They exercised.

And some of them pushed incredible boundaries. Professional distance runner Gabriele "Gabe" Grunewald received a rare cancer diagnosis with a poor long-term outlook—adenoid cystic carcinoma—in 2009, and then ran her fastest ever 1,500-hundred-meter race the next day. Despite setbacks and recurrences of her cancer, she continued training as an elite runner throughout treatment before passing away in 2019. (The ten-year overall survival of adenoid cystic carcinoma is 70 percent, lower with metastasis.) When I spoke to Gabe, she said, "My diagnosis was scary for me from the very beginning. But there were still things that I could do physically, and holding on to those things made me feel good. So using my body again, in a positive way, was very helpful—it gave me something to focus on one day at a time. From the very beginning, I feel like focusing on running has been a helpful coping mechanism. It's something that I can do today to improve my prognosis and improve my mood."

Renee Seman, a public defender from Long Island, New York, learned she had stage 4 breast cancer in 2014 and decided to set a goal of running all six of the most prestigious marathons in the world—New York, Chicago, Boston, Berlin, Tokyo, and London—a feat known as the Abbott World Marathon Majors. She completed her goal in 2019 (she did not run them all in one year), something only about 6,500 people in the world have done. "Running gives me time and a place to reflect, and deal with my emotions," she said in an article in *Runner's World.* "Running makes me feel good—it makes me feel capable. It gives me an opportunity to challenge my body. When I get into moods when I question, 'Why is my body revolting against me?' running makes me go, 'Oh well, I still have some control of my body.'"

The reason that so many caregivers and medical professionals have not embraced exercise during cancer treatment is because it's counterintuitive. It seems logical that exercise is tiring and that cancer would demand rest for your body to battle the disease. But here is the interesting thing that decades of research into exercise have taught us: The human body has evolved so that expending energy actually increases your energy. Your body is meant to be used—that is what makes it stronger. Being sedentary actually weakens your body. This holds true for cancer patients as well. Test it for yourself. Do you feel better sitting on the couch all day? Or getting out for a walk?

We've seen a similar mindset before with other health conditions, like heart disease. In the 1930s, if you had a heart attack, your doctor advised you to stay in bed for a full six weeks. Afterward, you were told to cut down your activity for the rest of your life. In the 1940s, a few pioneering cardiologists challenged this convention, and by the 1950s, the "cardiac chair" was introduced; patients were still resting, but upright. It took another twenty years for strong scientific evidence—including the Dallas Bed Rest and Training Study—to demonstrate the importance of exercise after a heart attack and the detrimental effects of prolonged bed rest. Early studies like this one provided the basis for developing an entire field—cardiac rehabilitation—dedicated to getting heart attack patients moving again. It's now firmly established that a patient should begin exercising as soon as possible after a heart attack. "In many cases doctors will recommend that survivors get more physical activity than they got before their heart attack," says the American Heart Association, and that "one of the best things you can do for yourself is to get into a cardiac rehabilitation program."

We see a similar trend in the advice historically given to women after delivering a baby and, more recently, in the way surgeons advise their patients during recovery from many operations. The conventional wisdom in both of these cases was to rest, but scientific evidence ultimately demonstrated—unequivocally—that moving, and moving as soon as possible, was clearly better.

HOW EXERCISE HELPS, SPECIFICALLY

As I've mentioned previously, the scientific evidence for exercise during cancer has reached a tipping point. Much like cardiac rehabilitation in the 1980s, there is a groundswell building—more and more of the medical establishment is beginning to accept that physical activity is not only beneficial for cancer patients, but that it should be a part of routine medical treatment.

Following are the areas in which we have the best evidence—where multiple studies have consistently shown that exercise provides a measurable and important benefit after a cancer diagnosis.

Anxiety. Regular aerobic exercise, and especially vigorous aerobic exercise or aerobic exercise combined with strength training, reduces the anxiety that many cancer patients feel after receiving the news that they have cancer and then throughout treatment. This has been shown across a number of the most common cancers, including breast, prostate, colorectal, and lung cancers, as well as blood cancers like leukemia, lymphoma, and myeloma. In general, studies have shown that the more vigorously you exercise, the less anxiety you feel.

Depression. Like anxiety, there are many trials that have clearly demonstrated that aerobic exercise reduces the depression patients often feel as they move through cancer treatment. Importantly, strength training alone doesn't seem to have a protective effect—you have to get up and move. Again, there may be what's known as a "dose-response" relationship between aerobic exercise and protection against depression—the more you exercise, the less depressed you feel.

Fatigue. The most counterintuitive benefit of exercise—the notion that forcing yourself to move when you are bone-tired will actually energize you—has some of the strongest evidence supporting it. Moderate-intensity aerobic exercise—aerobic exercise plus resistance training or resistance training alone—reduces fatigue both during and after treatment. Again counterintuitively, the harder you exercise, the less fatigue you are likely to feel. This also holds true for exercising longer than 30 minutes per session and carrying on your exercise program for more than three months.

However, fatigue does not have the same dose-response relationship as some other benefits of exercise. Right now, the scientific evidence shows that you really only need to get 90 minutes of exercise a week to see a significant benefit; you can go beyond that if you like, but it may not provide much more of a benefit. Finally, the boost in energy you get from regularly exercising is essentially the same whether you are doing it at home on your own or doing it in a supervised program or gym setting.

Health-related quality of life. This is a catchall term that researchers use to describe a person's overall physical and mental health. Scientific studies have consistently shown that exercise improves the way that people with cancer rate their overall health. This benefit has been shown across many different cancers, including breast, prostate, colorectal, lung, head and neck, bladder, and gynecological cancers, as well as blood cancers like lymphoma, leukemia, and myeloma. Combining aerobic exercise with resistance training seems to be more effective than either one alone.

Lymphedema. For many years, cancer patients who suffered this particular side effect of treatment—swelling that typically occurs in one of your arms or legs—were specifically told not to exercise. We now know conclusively, particularly for those with breast cancer, that resistance training using a "start low, progress slow" program of weight lifting is safe for women who either have or are at risk for developing lymphedema. It was my own research that turned the tide on this issue. Some studies suggest resistance training may help with preventing or improving lymphedema. Importantly, the strongest evidence has been in supervised weight-training programs, where an expert with training in exercise oncology or cancer rehabilitation can provide instruction.

While aerobic exercise seems to be safe and won't make lymphedema worse, we haven't focused these studies to prove that these kinds of workouts prevent or improve lymphedema. We also do not know whether the benefits we have seen in people with breast cancer extend to those with lymphedema from other types of cancers.

Physical function. When we talk about physical function in scientific studies, broadly speaking, what we mean is the ability to go about your daily life: shopping, cooking, cleaning, doing your job, and caring for yourself and your family. In scientific studies, we often use surveys and questionnaires to ask study participants how their cancer and treatment have affected their ability to do these activities so that we can get a good picture of whether they are able to go about their day-to-day lives. Many, many studies have shown that moderate-intensity aerobic training, resistance training, or combining both aerobic and resistance training improves cancer patients' physical function.

In the above six areas, we have really strong evidence that exercise leads to improvements. Dozens of studies from researchers at different clinics and medical institutions around the world show essentially the same thing: Exercise produces a noticeable benefit.

We also have evidence that exercise is beneficial in other areas; however, for one reason or another the evidence is not as strong. For example, there may be fewer studies or the studies may have a smaller number of patients included. Or perhaps there are a half dozen studies on a topic, but only five of the six show a benefit; the sixth one doesn't show any change as a result of exercising. What this means is that, taken as a whole, we still have good evidence for these benefits of exercise, but they are just not as strong as the ones outlined above.

Bone health. Most of the evidence for improving bone health during and after cancer treatment comes from studies of people with breast cancer or prostate cancer. In these studies, combining strength training with a high-impact activity such as jogging two or three times per week slowed bone loss or improved bone density. Importantly, regular aerobic training that was not high impact, like regular walking or riding a bicycle, did not have any effect on bone health. This is what we would expect based on similar studies done in people without cancer.

One other caveat is that we need more studies of cancer survivors with bone issues like osteoporosis. Right now, we're not sure whether higher-impact exercise is safe for these people, or what types might be most beneficial.

Sleep. There is mixed evidence on whether exercise leads to consistently better sleep during cancer treatment. Some studies have shown a small to moderate improvement in sleep quality from regular aerobic exercise; others have shown that exercise has no effect on sleep for those with cancer. However, in the general population there is very strong evidence that moderate to vigorous exercise leads to better sleep.

There are also a number of areas where evidence is *emerging* to prove whether exercise is helpful. We have a handful of studies that suggest there might be a benefit, but it would be irresponsible to say that we know this for sure.

Heart health. As cancer survivors live longer, they are beginning to experience all of the typical health concerns we associate with a long life, including heart disease. It is also well known that many cancer treatments damage the heart. Because of this, research on the heart health of cancer survivors is booming. There is promising—but early—research that exercise may protect against the damage caused by common cancer treatments. But these studies have not looked at the many different types of cancer or all of the different treatments. And of course, we do know that having a strong, well-functioning heart is a critical part of aging well, regardless of whether you have a cancer diagnosis in your history.

Nerve damage. Known as peripheral neuropathy, this common side effect of chemotherapy can cause weakness, numbness, and pain, usually in the hands and feet. When it is severe, it can affect balance and mobility. Right now we know that exercise is generally safe for people with cancer who are experiencing peripheral neuropathy; however, there are too few studies, and the results are too varied, to really understand whether and how much exercise helps.

Cognitive function. People undergoing cancer treatments—and not just chemotherapy, but also hormone therapy, radiation, and even surgery—may find they have difficulty remembering things, concentrating on tasks, or may simply experience a drop in overall mental "sharpness" after they've finished treatment. This is sometimes called "chemo brain" in the cancer community. Currently, there is some evidence in studies using animals that aerobic exercise can protect against changes to the brain that come with many cancer treatments. However, not a lot of studies have been done in humans, and those that have—primarily in women with breast cancer—have been inconsistent.

As with heart disease, we do know that exercise protects against the gradual decreases in memory, attention, and other forms of cognitive function typically seen in people as they grow older. It is likely—but not yet proven—that these same benefits will hold true for survivors of cancer as we do more research.

Nausea. In studies that have looked at a number of different benefits of exercise in people receiving chemotherapy, participants often say that exercise helped control their nausea. Still, there are no good studies looking specifically at nausea or at patients undergoing the chemotherapy treatments that are most likely to cause nausea. Again, there is some early research suggesting that exercise is helpful, but right now we cannot say this with certainty.

Pain. There is good, but not great, evidence that exercise helps with cancer pain. There are more studies in this area than some of the other side effects of treatment mentioned here, but they looked at the experience of pain in cancer patients overall, not specific kinds of pain, and most often they assessed this in studies that were really designed to look at something else first and foremost. That said, there have been well-done studies that have looked specifically at exercise for the pain caused by estrogen-blocking hormone therapy in women with breast cancer and shoulder pain in those with head and neck cancer. In both of these cases, exercise clearly helped. However, we need more studies like these focusing only on cancer-related pain.

Sexual function. Cancer dramatically affects a person's sex life—it's common but not often discussed. This is particularly true for cancers including breast cancer and prostate cancer that are driven by sex hormones like estrogen and testosterone. This is also true for cancers that require surgery near the sex organs, where unintended nerve damage could limit a person's sexual function.

Here the results have been mixed. Most of the research on exercise and sex has been done in men with prostate cancer, and while some studies have shown a benefit, others have not. In the general population, there is really good evidence that exercise improves your sex life; however, this side effect of cancer treatment is more complicated than some of the others discussed here. Many cancer treatments by their very nature act directly on hormones responsible for sex drive. Surgeries to remove cancer from the reproductive areas may damage nerves responsible for sensation during sex. That said, many cancer survivors continue to have active sex lives, and there is emerging evidence that exercise may help with this common side effect.

THIS BOOK RELIES ON SCIENCE FOR RECOMMENDATIONS

This is a book of the things we know work, based on medical research. It is based on research my colleagues and I have been doing for two decades or more. It is also based on personal experience, including the journey I've shared with my wife. But as an exercise scientist, I will not be recommending forms of exercise for which we do not have sufficient medical research to denote benefit. I can personally testify to the physical and mental well-being that different forms of exercise and movement provide. I have done tons of yoga and even more Pilates. But as an exercise scientist, I cannot say that these forms of exercise are supported by the same amount of medical research as aerobic and resistance exercise to benefit people living with and beyond cancer. I'm not saying they are not good; I am saying we do not have the same level of scientific evidence for them that we do for aerobic and resistance exercise.

INTERPRETING THE RESEARCH: WHAT'S TRUE?

Almost certainly at some point—and likely many points—throughout your cancer journey you will turn to the internet for answers about how you can help yourself during and after treatment. In some cases you will find helpful information. Dr. Liz O'Riordan, for example, told me that even as a breast cancer surgeon she found the advice she received from other breast cancer survivors she met on Twitter invaluable. They had simply figured out solutions unique to the experience of living with breast cancer that their oncologists had not. Many men with prostate cancer that I've met get incredibly helpful information from informal social networks, like family members or friends who have had the disease themselves.

However, there is also a lot of misinformation about cancer on the internet, which may also be repeated by well-meaning acquaintances. To help you discern what's credible from what's not, the remainder of this chapter is designed to help you evaluate health information, and in particular medical studies and evidence. This can be helpful when reading news about the latest cancer study online or even researching your unique cancer and its treatment online in databases like PubMed, the online archive of medical journals hosted by the National Institutes of Health's National Library of Medicine.

In the table below, we outline the characteristics of the three most common types of medical research conducted on cancer. *Basic science* refers to studies with genes, cells, and animals in a laboratory. These studies are tightly controlled, but the relevance of the findings to everyday patients is sometimes a stretch. *Clinical research* refers largely to randomized controlled trials with patients. These are the best type of evidence for this book, for your cancer journey. In these studies, scientists place

Table 2. Types of Medical Studies

	OBSERVATIONAL OR EXPERIMENTAL?	RANDOMIZED?	WHO DECIDES ON EXPOSURE?
Basic Science	Experimental	Sometimes	Scientist
Clinical Trials	Experimental	Usually	Scientist
Epidemiologic Studies	Observational	Never	Participant

patients into either an exercise or non-exercise group, using a process like flipping a coin (randomization). Patients are followed over time to discern whether the exercise treatments make a difference for the outcomes of interest, and then compare these differences to the group that did not get the exercise treatment.

This is very different from the third type of medical research, *epidemiologic studies*, in a few important ways. First, in an epidemiologic study, the participants are the ones who choose to be exposed to a risk factor or not. And the people who choose a given exposure are probably different in meaningful ways from those who choose not to be exposed (to smoking, for example). This could be important because it might be possible to conclude that the exposure of interest (smoking) is the cause of a disease or other outcome, when in fact it might be some other factor—for example, maybe the smokers also happen to live in homes with higher radon exposure, simply by chance. In a randomized controlled trial, the researchers choose who will be exposed, eliminating this possible source of confused results. In epidemiologic studies, the participants choose.

DONE WITH	SETTING	ADVANTAGES	DISADVANTAGES
Genes, cells, animals	Laboratory	Tight control	Questions about relevance to humans
Patients	Clinic	Randomization	Patients included may differ from average patient with condition under study
Patients/public	Community or clinic	More representative of the exposure in real life	Lack of control over unmeasured confounding variables

Another important difference is the dose of a given exposure. In a randomized controlled trial, the researcher chooses the amount of exposure. In epidemiologic studies, the participant chooses the amount of exposure. Despite these shortcomings, observational epidemiologic studies have been extraordinarily useful throughout history.

A good example of epidemiologic research at work is the case of cigarettes and lung cancer. It would be deeply unethical to do an experimental trial and ask one group of people to smoke and another to refrain and then see how they compare. (It would also take decades to complete, since the development of lung cancer is slow.) Instead, when researchers believed that cigarettes were causing lung cancer and needed to confirm it, they could look at the existing behavior of large groups of people—smokers and non-smokers—and make comparisons between them. Lung cancer is an obvious example, but epidemiologic studies are used to understand how a broad range of choices in our daily life affects our health.

The most important point to understand is the difference between *experimental evidence* and *observational evidence*. In an experimental study, the researchers are purposefully manipulating study participants' exposure to a medical intervention, and this is planned at the outset of the study, before patients even start receiving the treatment. In contrast, in an observational study, the researchers simply measure study participants' exposure to a medical intervention or lifestyle factor (like smoking, exercise, or a certain diet). In other words, participants in observational studies are going about their lives and researchers are simply observing them to see how different lifestyle choices or medical treatments are affecting them. Once they have large enough groups that have made these unique choices, they can compare them.

This difference gets to the heart of interpreting health studies: causality, or the relationship between a suspected cause and an effect. Splashy headlines online often tout the results of medical studies as being much more definitive than they really are. Some common ones include saying that drinking coffee or eating a particular food causes people to live longer (or die younger). Almost invariably, these studies are observational; they have simply demonstrated that many people who live long lives also drink coffee—it could be that people who drink coffee also tend to exercise more, and that is why they live longer.

To truly determine a cause-and-effect relationship, researchers need to establish a number of things. First, the exposure must occur before the outcome of interest. For example, to show that exercise reduces fatigue in cancer patients, the exercise must occur before any change in fatigue. In addition, the relationship must be plausible, meaning there should be a reasonable biological explanation for why the two things being measured are associated. It must also be strong—that is, the exposure must result in robust changes in the outcome. It must also be consistent; experiments done by different researchers in different places and at different times should produce similar results. It should also be specific—there should be no other likely explanation. And there should be a dose-response relationship; greater exposure to the intervention in question should lead to a greater incidence of the effect.

There are other criteria, as well, and establishing a reliable cause-and-effect relationship in medicine takes years, even decades. Given all of this, how do we actually know when something is proven? When we have what my mentor Dr. Henry Blackburn called "the three beauties": evidence from each of the types of medical studies outlined above—basic science studies, clinical studies, and epidemiologic studies. When all three of these are working in concert—when results of each of them support the other two—we can really say, "OK, now we have something."

As you look at medical information online and elsewhere, here are a few other factors to consider.

Animal studies. Cancer has been "cured" countless times in studies of drugs in animals. Only very rarely do these supposedly miracle cures even make it into drug trials with human patients; of those that do eventually get tested in patients, only a fraction are safe and effective enough to be used widely. If you see a headline touting something that appears miraculous or overblown in a study using animals, it will be many years, or even decades, before that treatment makes its way to humans.

Significance. Reports of health studies often talk about "statistical significance." What this measures, simply, is the degree to which a given relationship between two things is likely not caused by chance. The likelihood that something will be "statistically significant" depends on the number of participants in the study as well as the strength of the effect. In very large studies, it is easy to see effects that are statistically significant; however, a statistically significant result does not necessarily mean that it is significant to you as a patient. If you have a large group of people experiencing pain after surgery and each ranked their pain as a 10 on a scale of 1 to 10—meaning very severe—and a brand-new pain reliever reduces that score to a 9 for most of them, you may have a "statistically significant" relationship between the pain score and the drug in question. But these patients are still experiencing a 9 level of pain! If patients need to get down to a 6 or 7 to get out of bed and carry on with life, then reducing the pain by one point does not particularly matter, even if the results of the study are "statistically significant."

You may also fall into the group of people for whom the pain reliever doesn't work at all. Or worse, the pain reliever might also cause gastrointestinal problems, perhaps far worse problems than the issue it is supposed to solve.

For all of these reasons, "statistical significance" should not be interpreted to mean that something has been proven helpful to patients in a meaningful way.

Bias. This is anything that causes the results of a medical study to deviate from the truth. There are many forms of bias, including the way that a medical study is designed or the manner in which its results are interpreted. But one of the most basic checks for bias you can do is to think about whether the person presenting the information has a financial interest at stake. If the study you are reading about a food was funded by its manufacturer, you should be more skeptical of the results. If the article that you are reading on the anticancer benefits of a particular supplement is presented on a website that sells alternative medicines—or receives advertising dollars from companies that make alternative medicines—then you should be very critical of any information being presented. Bias can be incredibly difficult to assess. The most important point is to think critically about health information before you assume that what you are reading or hearing is accurate.

I've spent the last few pages of this chapter talking about health studies and scientific evidence not only because there is so much misinformation on the internet, on television, and in all the other different media we consume, but also because I want you to know that I'm only putting information into this book that meets the high scientific standards outlined earlier. The benefits of exercise that I've mentioned here—reducing anxiety, depression, fatigue, and lymphedema and improving physical function and quality of life, among others—have all passed rigorous assessments of consistency, validity, strength, plausibility, and other criteria to determine a true cause-and-effect relationship. We have evidence from basic science experiments done in laboratories, from individual patients in clinics, and from large databases all pointing in the same direction: Exercise causes these desired effects during and after cancer treatment. And when I discuss something that does not meet this high standard, you will know because I will point out that it is emerging science or promising research—these are positive effects of exercise for people with cancer that we hope to confirm in the coming years.

FINDING MOTIVATION

Kikkan Randall was devastated. She was twenty-eight days into treatment and deep into her second round of chemo, and she could barely speak above a whisper. She was feverish and exhausted. Exercise was absolutely out of the question.

If anyone should have been able to handle breast cancer treatment, it was Kikkan. A mere six months prior, with teammate Jessie Diggins, she had become the first US athlete to win Olympic gold in cross-country skiing, a notoriously difficult sport that demands exceptionally high levels of endurance, strength, and speed. The duo's photo finish, in which Diggins narrowly edged out perennial powerhouse Sweden, captured the nation's attention in a sport that few were familiar with.

Three months after her gold medal–winning performance, Kikkan received the news that she had stage 2B breast cancer while en route to a friend's wedding. She was in the shape of her life and even though she retired shortly after her Olympic win, she had plans to keep up a rigorous schedule of mountain biking, running, and gym workouts twice a week. "When I got the diagnosis, my first reaction was, 'I'm just going to keep doing what I can,'" Kikkan told me. "I just made the rule that I would follow my body. If I felt good, I would do what I had planned. And if not, I was always able to back down."

Ultimately, successive rounds of chemo took their toll on her. "The best way to describe it is that it's a general flu-like feeling. The chemo drugs definitely messed with my gastrointestinal system. And with the fatigue, I was sleeping extra or just kind of lying around. It also affected my mental state—I just didn't feel super motivated or clearly focused. And as the chemo went on progressively, I had a heavy feeling in my legs, the kind I experienced during my career when I was really training a lot."

Even world-class athletes, who have found the motivation to exercise day in and day out for decades, have bad days in treatment, where they simply can't find the motivation or the energy to exercise.

Almost certainly there is going to come a time during treatment—perhaps for some it will be the *entire* treatment—when you are going to say, "I don't want to exercise." Even if you have the desire to get up and move, even just to walk to the mailbox at the end of the driveway, you may feel like you simply cannot muster the strength.

Many people say that you don't really know what fatigue is until you've had cancer. It is often described as the most common, most debilitating side effect of cancer treatment.

It can be shocking just how deeply fatigued you feel during cancer treatment. Some people talk about "living life at half energy." Those who work through treatment may find they have to cut their days to half-time, from eight hours to four. Even then, they still find they are just as tired after a four-hour day as they were after a full eight-hour one prior to treatment. A walk at half speed, or half the typical distance, leaves you just as tired as your regular one.

As Kikkan told me, it is not limited to physical energy either. Cancer fatigue also affects your mental state. It is common during cancer treatment to feel like you simply cannot concentrate. Formerly simple activities, like reading a book, may become too difficult to enjoy.

It is important to understand that cancer fatigue is not merely severe tiredness. It is very different from the tiredness you feel after pulling an all-nighter to study for an exam or even the kind of chronic exhaustion you feel from working too many hours and not sleeping enough for weeks on end. For many people with cancer, sleeping more doesn't help their fatigue. In fact, many people with cancer fatigue don't have the desire to sleep more, which is quite different from feeling tired, where all you want to do is crawl into bed.

Another key difference is that researchers don't completely know what causes cancer fatigue, despite the fact that it is incredibly common. In many patients, it can be caused by an inflammatory response to the treatments used against cancer. In some advanced cancer patients, it may be caused by cancer itself. It is possible that fatigue is caused by injury to your normal, noncancerous cells during treatment or possibly from your body's efforts to repair damage by treatments to healthy cells and tissue. It may come on gradually over time or start suddenly. It may last only for the duration of treatment or extend beyond treatment for months, years, or even the remainder of your life.

Given this level of fatigue—which many patients describe as the most exhausted feeling imaginable, the sense that you cannot even lift your head from the pillow—how can anyone be expected to move, let alone exercise?

While moving more seems counterproductive at first glance, exercise is the number-one recommended treatment for cancer fatigue in the most widely used treatment guidelines for cancer, which are published by the National Comprehensive Cancer Network and used daily by oncologists in their clinics.

This recommendation is based on the results of more than 200 studies looking at the effects of exercise on cancer fatigue. As just one example, a recent study in Australia randomly assigned a group of 163 prostate cancer patients to one of three groups: The first did strength training and body-weight exercises like bounding, skipping, and jumping; the second did strength training plus aerobic exercise like walking, jogging, cycling, and rowing; and the third group served as the study "control" and did not change anything about their usual treatments or activities. The researchers then checked in on the patients both six months and a year later.

The study had two very important findings: First, all of the different exercise programs reduced fatigue and improved vitality; and second, those with the highest levels of fatigue and lowest vitality when the study started improved the most with exercise.

Many other studies have come to similar conclusions. In another one published in 2017, researchers combined data from 113 similar studies, ultimately including more than 11,525 people with cancer, that measured the effects of exercise on fatigue. In this analysis, notably, the comparison was made between effects of pharmacologic, or drug, interventions versus exercise interventions for cancer fatigue. Again, in this very large group of people with cancer, regular exercise improved fatigue both during and following cancer treatment by as much as 30 percent—a very significant improvement and quite possibly the difference between taking control of your fatigue and being controlled by it. But the take-home message is that drug interventions did not have any measurable effect on fatigue. What I'm telling you is that there is not a drug on the market more effective for your cancer-related fatigue than exercise.

Knowing that fatigue is the most common side effect of cancer treatment—affecting between 50 and 95 percent of patients depending on the type of cancer and treatment—the question becomes: How do you get past it to experience the benefits of exercise?

Perhaps the most important thing to understand is that when it comes to finding the motivation to get up and move, you are the expert. Only you know what motivates you and what will drive you to get it done. And there is not one approach that motivates everyone; our motivations are unique to each of us, and they even vary over time and from situation to situation. The studies I've mentioned above are good because they convincingly demonstrate that exercise is the best treatment we have for fatigue, but all the studies in the world are unlikely to get anyone out the door and moving. Our personal desires are what motivate us to do this; we are driven by the things that matter to us—feeling well enough to attend and enjoy an upcoming wedding, wanting to spend time with a grandchild, or wanting to be there for the people who rely on us.

A cancer diagnosis is life changing; it's what physicians and behavioral psychologists call a "teachable moment." But a better way to think about it is that it's a *motivational moment*. When you're faced with a cancer diagnosis, it becomes crystal clear what matters to you in life. And that can become your motivation.

As you read this chapter, ask yourself: On a scale of 1 to 10, how confident am I that I am going to do what is recommended in this book? If you are already in treatment, then change the question slightly: How confident am I that I'm going to get my exercise done this week?

It's very important to be honest with yourself. There is no one watching or judging you. Getting up and moving regularly—especially while you are dealing with a cancer diagnosis and treatment—is incredibly hard! As we know from stories like Kikkan's, even people who love to exercise and do it for a living have moments during their treatment when they find it incredibly difficult.

If on a scale of 1 to 10, the answer is 2, then the question becomes, What would it take for it to be a 7 or an 8? Let your mind wander. There are no right or wrong answers to these questions. For some, the answer to this one might be emotional, like remembering that you need to exercise to be as healthy as you can for a big upcoming life event or milestone. For others, the answer could be logistical: You need to buy new running shoes. You need to make sure that you have a safe place to exercise. You need somebody to exercise with you. You need to rearrange your schedule to be free for the exercise class you really enjoy taking.

Write these down. And write down the fears or aspirations that drove you to pick up this book in the first place. Really think about the steps, no matter how small, that would make your answer of a 2 to the question above an 8 instead. List them all.

Perhaps you already move pretty regularly. Or you are at a place in your cancer journey where you are able to exercise regularly. In this case, perhaps you're at an 8 already. Write down the things that have been important for you to get that regular exercise. Again, they can be emotional or aspirational, like "I feel better when I exercise" or "On days I move more, I know I'm doing my best to take care of myself." Or they may be completely logistical, like "It's easier to get my exercise in when I do it in the morning instead of waiting until the afternoon."

The effort that you put in now, thinking about why you want to exercise and what will help you get there, will be incredibly important throughout your journey.

Simply having a list at the end of this process is very helpful, but it also matters *how* you approach making this list—a technique known as motivational interviewing. Like everything else in this book, the process of finding your motivation to exercise is based on science, in this case the field of behavioral science, which studies why we act the way we do and how we can make lasting changes for the better in our daily lives.

Motivational interviewing—in which you talk about why you want to change and what it would take to make changes in your life—is well studied and recognized as one of the most effective ways to change your habits. People are best motivated to change when they themselves discover their reasons to change.

Making a physical list, even if it's stored on your phone or digitally somewhere else, is an important part of the process. In doing this, you are hearing yourself think about change and then saying it aloud by putting it down in words. This is known as "change talk," and the more we hear ourselves talk about change, the more motivated we are to actually change.

It is also important because most of the time there will not be anyone guiding you—or motivating you—to exercise. At some points, you might get brief guidance from a surgeon or your oncologist, or see a physical therapist, but for the most part you will be guiding and motivating yourself to exercise throughout treatment. Really thinking through your reasons for doing this, and figuring out what it will take for you to do it day in and day out, will help cement your motivation.

Once you have figured out your motivation, there are a few practical steps that you can take to keep it up. By following them, you are more likely to stick to your resolution to get up and move.

The "10 minute" rule. Nearly all of the cancer patients I speak with who keep up their exercise routine during and after treatment use this rule in some form. This approach to exercising during cancer treatment has been tried and tested by so many patients that even though it has never been formally studied in a research trial, it has been almost universally accepted by exercise scientists.

It's incredibly straightforward: Start exercising, and if after 10 minutes you feel better, keep going. If you feel worse after 10 minutes, stop. More often than not, you will want to keep going.

Keep a log. As we mentioned in chapter 2, creating an activity log is one of the first and most important steps you'll take while training during treatment. It is a simple way to keep track of what you did on a given day and how it made you feel.

The log is not meant for you to look back on your achievements— though you should do that from time to time—but rather to help you *look forward*. The real value of a log is in recognizing trends, and in particular the way that cancer and cancer treatments are affecting your activities and the way you feel afterward. For example, once you are in the midst of treatment, you'll begin to recognize the difference between a 10-minute walk done the day after a chemotherapy infusion versus a walk four days after an infusion. It will also help you establish "a new normal" each time your cancer journey takes a turn, such as the start of hormonal treatments or radiotherapy, and help you recognize when things "feel off" and you should *conserve* your energy rather than risk overtraining. This will help you recognize what Dr. Liz O'Riordan called her "bad days."

The next chapter introduces the first training program and includes the elements to list in your daily log. Chapter 2 provided a simple format to follow (blank forms are downloadable from www.movingthrough cancer.com).

Use SMART goals. Countless organizations have used this approach to help individuals achieve their goals. Very simply, SMART goals are:

- **Specific:** Improvement in a particular area or skill

- **Measurable:** Include some way to indicate or suggest progress

- **Achievable:** Can be accomplished under the expected circumstances

- **Relevant:** Worthwhile and applicable

- **Time-bound:** Have a deadline, whether that be one day or a period of months

Setting your exercise goals using these criteria can be really helpful for reducing any anxiety you might have about exercising. Rather than seeing a six-month or yearlong stretch of effort ahead of you, it really encourages you to break down your goals into manageable pieces. They can be as small as the exercises you hope to do today, or simply the practical steps you need to take—such as setting out your tennis shoes or workout clothes—to make exercising more likely.

It also provides a sense of accomplishment—it feels good to tick goals off your to-do list, and setting small, achievable goals builds a sense of accomplishment into your regular exercise. And of course, as with writing down your motivations, formally setting goals makes you more likely to achieve them.

Do something you enjoy. Throughout this book, I'm going to provide a number of different exercise programs based on the best available scientific evidence, each one designed to help at specific points before, during, and after cancer treatment. While these programs are based on proven results, it is very important not to get stuck on the idea that if you can't do exactly what is recommended, then it's not worth doing at all. That would ignore one of the most important truths in exercise science: that doing some movement, even every once in a while, is much better than not doing anything. In other words, a little is a lot more than nothing.

Everything counts. Any kind of activity or movement is better than sitting and will translate into some benefit. No one, including you, benefits from sitting on the couch all day for days on end. There have only been a few exercise science studies that have evaluated gardening as a form of physical activity; that said, anyone who has spent an afternoon planting or weeding knows that it is physical work. And all physical work that you do during cancer treatment will improve your fitness on some level.

Social support. Exercising with a friend has many benefits. When researchers at the Institute of Sport, Exercise and Active Living in Melbourne, Australia, summarized the results of twenty-seven published studies, they found that people were much more likely to exercise when they did so with another person, and that this effect was even stronger when the other person was a family member. It also feels better to exercise with another person. Those who exercise with a friend report that the experience is more calming; other studies have found that exercising in groups reduces stress and increases mental and emotional well-being compared with exercising alone. Finally, people tend to exercise more vigorously when they're with someone else, particularly when the other person is more fit, due to a behavioral phenomenon known as the Kohler effect—no one wants to be the slowest or weakest person in a group, so everyone works harder as a result.

Get out into nature. It is not surprising that disconnecting from our busy lives and getting outside into nature—a practice known in Japan as "forest bathing"—is good for us. We know intuitively that it feels good, but recently researchers have done many studies comparing indoor versus outdoor exercise to understand why. Not surprisingly, exercising outdoors feels more revitalizing, engaging, and satisfying than being indoors, and when people exercise outdoors they feel more committed to doing it again later. Exercising outdoors also seems to improve self-esteem and reduce tension, anger, and depression—common feelings immediately after a cancer diagnosis. Interestingly, the first five minutes of exercising outdoors appears to have the biggest impact on mood and self-esteem.

There are even research studies suggesting that exercising outside feels easier than exercising indoors. When researchers track walking speed, those exercising outdoors tend to walk faster, even though, paradoxically, they actually report that they're exerting less effort in doing so.

Revisit your motivations. Without question, at some point during treatment your motivation to get up and exercise will drop. This is entirely normal; it's even expected. It's not a reason to beat yourself up or feel bad. But it is a reason to revisit the list of motivations you wrote earlier in this chapter. In moments where you are not feeling motivated, go back to this list to remember why you have committed to exercising and review any simple steps you can take to help you get it done.

There are a couple of larger truths in medicine that we've learned and that may be helpful when it comes to maintaining your motivation to exercise, despite all of the fatigue, both physical and emotional, that comes with cancer.

The first is this: At the end of the day, the best exercise program is the one that you will do. And that is likely to be the one you enjoy the most. This is a key message of *Moving Through Cancer*, and one that will be repeated throughout: Move. And keeping moving in whatever way works for you.

Dr. Bill Kraus is a friend and colleague who serves as the director of the Duke Rehabilitation Program at Duke University. Dr. Kraus has spent his professional life studying how exercise lowers the risk of a heart attack. When I spoke with him, he put it very simply: "It turns out that everything counts. The point is that anything is better than sitting and is going to translate into some benefit."

He advocates a "glass half full" approach. If your target is to take an extra 2,000 steps per day and you only get to 1,000, you may look at that as a failure—you didn't hit your goal. But looked at another way, Dr. Kraus points out that by taking those extra 1,000 steps, you have already done more than 90 percent of the US population to improve your health! That's an important realignment of perspective, particularly if you're playing the "long game" of improving your health over the course of months or even years of cancer treatment and many years as a cancer survivor.

But it need not be walking, even though that's the most commonly studied and prescribed exercise for cancer patients. You can jump on a mini-trampoline, ride your bike, take a class at the local gym, or go ballroom dancing with your partner—at the end of the day, getting your heart rate up is all that matters, regardless of how you do so.

That leads to the second larger truth: The benefits of exercise are most significant in the transition from doing nothing to doing something. If you take a marathon runner and add an additional 10 minutes of exercise to their daily training schedule, that extra 10 minutes is not going to make much of a difference. But for someone who has not been to the gym or exercised in several years, 10 additional minutes of exercise per day is going to have very significant and measurable effects on their overall health and well-being. The following graph, taken from a 1994 publication by Dr. William Haskell, nicely sums up this well-established evidence.

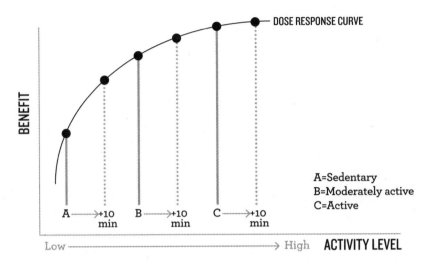

Exercise Dose Response Curve: Small Changes Matter

The vertical axis shows the benefit of more activity. The higher this is, the better. The horizontal axis shows the benefit from increasing physical activity a small amount, say 10 minutes a day. Notice that there are three groups labeled A for sedentary, B for moderately active, and C for most active. Then notice that the improvement in physical benefit from increasing activity by 10 minutes a day is greatest among the sedentary group. Then look further out to the right, to the benefit of adding 10 minutes of exercise a day among the most active. The benefit is negligible.

This information is very important to remember, particularly on days when you are not feeling motivated to do your full planned workout: The benefits of exercise are gained most in the transition from nothing to something.

Put another way: Please do not get stuck on the idea that if you cannot exactly follow the programs outlined in this book the entire time you are going through treatment, then it's not worth doing at all. The truth is that if you can do something, even just every once in a while, you are still going to be much better off than if you did nothing at all. We are not asking you to run. We are asking you to stand up and take a walk—even if your first walk is just to the mailbox.

PART TWO

THE MOVING THROUGH CANCER PROGRAM

PREHABILITATION
(TRAINING BEFORE TREATMENT)

ancer affects everyone differently, and I see many different reactions in the people who come through the cancer clinic. But time and again, the ones who thrive, rather than just survive, are those who play an active role in their treatment. They are trying to beat their cancer, and they're also trying to live their best life. Cancer warrior Gabe Grunewald had an Albert Einstein quote over her couch: "There are only two ways to live your life. One is as though nothing is a miracle. The other is as though everything is a miracle."

The time before you start treatment is a window of opportunity. It's a chance to get in the shape of your life for the fight of your life. And during a time when you may feel out of control, exercise is a way to retake some control.

When Dr. Liz O'Riordan, the breast cancer surgeon, was diagnosed with breast cancer herself at the age of forty, none of the doctors she saw for her diagnosis and treatment suggested that she exercise. But staying active was one of the most empowering things she could do. "For me, exercise is about cancer not defining me. I wasn't going to let cancer take everything away from me," she said. "And just being outside in the fresh air training made me think only about training. I wasn't thinking about the fact that I had cancer. I was just enjoying being alive."

This is one of the greatest benefits of exercise during the extremely stressful and difficult period between a cancer diagnosis and the start of treatment—it empowers you and takes your mind off cancer at the same time.

You don't need to be a world-class athlete to reap these benefits. Even if you've been living a mostly sedentary life and have as little as two weeks before cancer treatment begins, you can still get important benefits from starting a regular exercise program now.

THE EVIDENCE FOR EXERCISE BEFORE TREATMENT BEGINS

Your doctors may not be aware of the evidence supporting exercise before starting cancer treatment. However, there is more and more research being published each year suggesting that they should recommend exercise routinely.

There are now dozens of scientifically rigorous studies on exercise before cancer treatment that show a program of training for treatment has significant, measurable, and important benefits for patients. The name for such interventions is "prehabilitation," denoting it is the opposite of "rehabilitation." For prehabilitation, the goal is to improve your physical and emotional well-being *before* treatment starts. The patients who engage in prehabilitation (training before treatment) are stronger, healthier, happier, and better prepared for the next phase of their life, whether that's additional treatments or life as a cancer survivor.

As just one example, take a look at the following figure from recent research published by two of the leading minds in this field, Dr. Daniel Santa Mina and Dr. Francesco Carli. Two groups of prostate cancer patients about to start treatment with surgery were studied: One group did 60 minutes of moderate exercise at home using resistance bands, a stability ball, and a yoga mat three to four days a week; the other group—the "control" group—was given a handout listing exercises to train only the pelvic floor muscles, which help control urination and sexual function, and are considered "usual care" for all men undergoing prostate surgery.

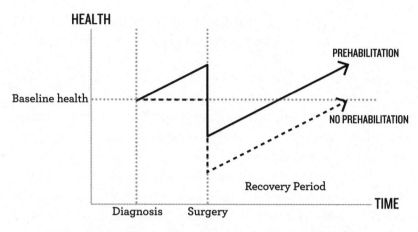

Trajectory of Health Parameters with and without Prehabilitation

The results of the study showed that patients who exercised could walk faster and longer, were stronger and slimmer, and had less anxiety throughout their treatment. These differences showed up as early as the day of surgery and continued to be seen as late as six months after surgery, the furthest time point researchers measured. Importantly, as shown in the figure, they recovered from surgery more quickly, allowing them to get back to their routine life much faster.

The results of this randomized, controlled trial are echoed in larger studies that have looked not at specific training regimens, but rather at overall physical activity among much larger groups of people with cancer. For example, in one study that looked at exercise in more than 49,000 patients with either breast or colorectal cancer, those who started exercising after they were diagnosed were more likely to survive their disease.

These positive changes can also happen very quickly. When my wife, Sara, was diagnosed, her oncologist told her, "You have aggressive cancer in your nose; see you in four weeks." That was it! That's all we were given in terms of how to prepare for treatment, and this is a common experience. But the body adapts to training quickly, and fitness can improve in just a handful of exercise sessions. It doesn't matter whether you only have a week before your treatment begins; there is evidence that you can do yourself some good.

WHAT IS THE GOAL OF TRAINING
BEFORE TREATMENT?

As you'll learn throughout this book, different stages of the fight against cancer require different approaches to training. You will feel very differently depending on what treatment, and how many of those treatments, you have received. And you will also be training specifically to counteract the negative side effects of the treatment that is next for you or currently underway.

When you are training before treatment, the focus is on gaining and maintaining muscle mass. To be clear, the goal is not necessarily to increase strength, though there is a natural parallel between muscle mass and strength, and increases in strength will happen as a result of increasing muscle mass.

Muscle is a "use it or lose it" tissue that atrophies—or disappears, more or less—if it is not used. In short, it's "expensive" to the body in terms of nutrients and energy to maintain, so if it's not being used, the body will not keep it around. When treatment starts, it is almost certain that your activity levels will go down, at least some. In the case of surgery, your activity level may go down to zero during the initial recovery. During this period, your body will shed muscle to conserve energy. Having more muscle mass at the beginning of treatment means there will be more around at the end, when you've recovered from this initial treatment and must be ready to start additional, new forms of treatment.

The mindset of training before treatment is to focus on your healthy cells. During a typical cancer treatment, the focus is usually on the cancer cells, the ones that are working against you. It's important for your medical team to focus on your cancer in order to eliminate it, but that perspective ignores the trillions of healthy cells—the overwhelming majority in your body, in fact—that are there to help during cancer treatment. These are the cells we're focusing on when we talk about training for treatment. They are genetically programmed to help you, but their ability to do so depends on how much energy is left over after getting through the daily work of breathing, digesting, moving around, dressing, working, caring for yourself and your family, and however else you spend your time.

As an example, let's say you are the average American—you can get through the day without much trouble, but if you need to work harder physically, like taking a hike or chasing a grandchild, you'll be pretty tired by the end of the day, or even need an afternoon nap. Let's make up a system of work units to describe what happens to your fitness during treatment. If 100 is an Olympic athlete, let's say you are a 30. And let's assume that it takes 20 units to get through your day, but that it takes an additional 20 units of energy to get through cancer treatment. You need 40 units to get through every day—but you only have 30. That means that every day you are going to be at an energy deficit and really wiped out during treatment. That will make it hard to keep working. And it will make it hard to continue caring for yourself. And, since you are working beyond your capacity, the ability of your healthy cells to help is impaired—they do not have the energy. Further, you will move less, you will lose muscle mass and aerobic fitness, and you will finish treatment more depleted than when you went in. Then, instead of being a 30, you are closer to a 20, maybe even a 10. Getting back to 30 will feel really hard.

The lesson: Even the ability to complete a normal day in the life of a typical American will be hard after the additional challenges of cancer treatment. Increasing your muscle mass and energy reserves beforehand will help prevent the losses in fitness and everyday function that are typically seen during cancer treatment.

Now, let's say that you spend six weeks working out consistently before entering cancer treatment and you get to a fitness/energy level of 50. Twenty of these go to daily activities and an additional 20 go to recovering from cancer treatment. That means you have a bit of capacity left over and available to your body. Your healthy cells now have an improved ability to contribute to healing after treatment, such as taming inflammation or fighting infection.

Again, before treatment begins, resistance exercise is the number-one priority. Resistance exercise means making your muscles work against a weight or opposing force. And the goal is to maintain and even gain muscle, which is not necessarily the same as gaining and maintaining strength.

The window of time before you begin treatment is your chance to be in control of your narrative and your body for the last time in a while. So hit it! This is the time!

GETTING STARTED

Here is a program to begin regularly exercising and prepare for cancer treatment, whether that is surgery, chemotherapy (or other drug treatments), or radiation. The program makes some assumptions. First, that you are currently not working out much. If you're getting regular exercise, gauge what you are currently doing against what we recommend in the pages that follow. Increase what you are doing by approximately 10 percent, or add the missing elements. For example, if you take a daily walk but you have not lifted weights before, keep walking and add the weight-lifting portion of the program. If you currently lift twice a week, add a third session per week. Approach what you see in the following sections from the perspective that you are *training for treatment*. Exercise is meant to push your body and leave you feeling a bit out of breath. But also note that training so hard that you hurt yourself is counterproductive. Listen to your body and back off if it's telling you you're doing too much.

If you can find a certified fitness professional to help you, please do. And if the program isn't working for you, and you would prefer to do a fitness class or a high-intensity interval training class at the local gym, go! The point is this: Do more than you've been doing.

Second, as an example, the program assumes you have exactly twenty-one days until treatment begins. If you have less time, start at twenty-one days and do what you can until the day your treatment begins. If you have more time, do some days twice, or progress to "T minus 2 days until treatment" (page 76) and keep doing that workout until your first day of treatment. It's your journey.

THE PROGRAM:
TRAINING BEFORE TREATMENT

The program for training before treatment focuses on five areas: log, move, lift, eat, and sleep. Before treatment, the priority is lift. You want to maintain—and even gain—as much muscle mass as possible before your treatment starts. Lifting weights is the best way to achieve this.

The log, move, eat, and sleep components will support lift during your training for treatment. You will do them every day, and for the most part, they remain the same throughout this phase of training. But do not underestimate them: They're critical for supporting your body and getting the best results from the lift program.

LOG

You'll want to start logging what you are doing and how you are feeling before your treatment starts. This will provide a baseline to help you know how treatment is changing your ability to exercise and your response to exercising. Again, the log is meant to help you *look forward*. Its real value is in recognizing trends and understanding the way that cancer and cancer treatments are affecting your activities and the way you feel afterward. For example, once you are in the midst of treatment, you'll begin to recognize the difference between a 10-minute walk the day after a chemotherapy infusion versus four days after one. It will also help you establish "a new normal" each time you finish or start a new treatment and help you recognize when things "feel off" and you should *conserve* your energy rather than risk overdoing it.

Get in the habit now of using a log to record your move, lift, eat, and sleep habits. As mentioned in chapter 2, you can make this like a log or more like a star chart. This is something your family can do for you, if you like. For blank downloadable charts, see chapter 2 or my website, www.movingthroughcancer.com.

You can, of course, include other items, particularly if you find them relevant to how you feel during your activities or if they make tracking your energy levels easier. For example, it can be helpful to give your activity session a simple letter grade based on how you felt during and immediately after the session.

A: I am superhuman!
B: Good workout
C: I felt fatigued
D: Shortened or otherwise modified activity
E: Couldn't complete activity

If you start seeing three or more Cs or Ds showing up in a row, that suggests it is time to dial back your intensity and conserve a bit more energy, rather than risk overtraining and depleting yourself.

You could choose to include perceived effort on your log too, which is the most useful way to measure your effort before and during cancer treatment. (Other measures, like heart rate, can become unreliable once you start treatments like chemotherapy.) Perceived effort uses a simple 1 to 10 scale, where 1 is sitting on the couch with the remote in hand and 10 is running as fast as you can, like to catch a bus or a plane.

Another way to think of exercise intensity is using the "breath test." For light activities, you should be able to breathe through your nose only. Moderate activities are done at a "conversational pace"; you can talk in complete sentences, but you cannot sing. At a vigorous level of activity, you have trouble talking and may be out of breath.

When logging your activity, it is not so important what a 4 or a 6 is for you; in fact, a 4 for one person may feel quite different for someone else. The most important thing is that you remain consistent with your own grading. Over time, this simple scale will become very accurate for gauging how an activity made you feel on a given day.

Don't allow what we're recommending to add to your anxiety. This is a very busy time, one that may include organizing childcare, eldercare, job responsibilities, and many other tasks you may not be able to get to for a while. It's like the holiday season, but in this case it's all of the extra work without any of the joy. There is stress naturally during this time and what we're recommending should reduce your stress. If it is increasing it, back off.

(X) MOVE

Walk, run, bike, dance, or swim for at least 30 minutes each day. Make sure that you are breathing more heavily than usual but not gasping for air. Follow the "talk but not sing" rule: You should be able to talk but not be able to hold a note (regardless of your singing ability). If you can't talk, you are working too hard. If you can sing, you are not working hard enough.

Each day, try to add a little bit more. If you did 20 minutes yesterday, shoot for 21 or 22 today, and then 23 or 24 the next. As your body allows, continue progressively adding more time and intensity during your move session each day.

(🏋) LIFT

Throughout the lift program, you will be doing five exercises. These are the core movements of the lift program. After a day off to assess your body's response, you will add more repetitions or resistance to each set. Videos explaining each of these exercises and videos to follow along as you do these exercises can be found at www.movingthroughcancer.com. The recommended exercises are described on the following pages.

CHEST PRESS

Lie on your back on a weight-lifting bench, an aerobic step, or on the floor on a towel. Starting with arms straight, bend your elbows to right angles, elbows away from the body, then return arms to straight over your chest. When you add resistance, this will become challenging.

START 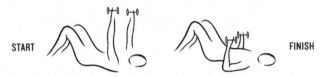 FINISH

ONE-ARM ROW

Place one knee and one hand on a chair or the edge of the bed, as shown in the illustrations. Start with your free hand hanging down. Squeeze your shoulder blade toward your spine as you bend your elbow to raise your fist toward your side. Slowly lower to the starting position. Switch and do the other side.

START 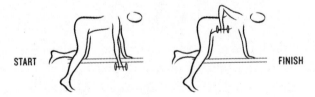 FINISH

SQUATS

Stand in front of a full-length mirror, facing to the side. Feet should be hip distance apart with toes pointing forward. Hold your weights at your sides (like suitcases), as shown. Sit backward like you are going to sit down in a chair, keeping your chest lifted, eyes forward. In fact, to start, keep a chair behind you, so that if you touch the chair, you will know you've gone down far enough. Sneak a peek at your knees in a mirror: They shouldn't bend past 90 degrees. Sneak a peek at your knees by looking down: Your knees should not go out past your toes and should stay parallel (not drift toward or away from each other).

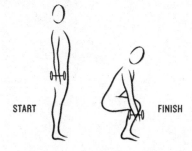

START   FINISH

LUNGES

Hold on to a chair or the wall and step backward with one foot so that you can bend both knees to 90-degree angles, while keeping your chest up. Return to the starting position. Repeat for a full set on one side before switching to the other leg. If you can do lunges without holding on, that's great too. To add resistance for the supported lunge, hold on with one hand and hold a weight in the other hand, at your side.

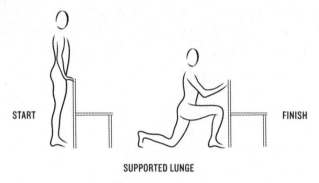

START   FINISH

SUPPORTED LUNGE

DEADLIFTS

Stand with your feet hip-width apart. Bend just at the hips, letting the head follow the back so you are looking at the floor at the end of the movement. Return to standing.

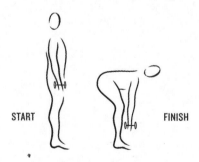

START   FINISH

(✗) EAT

Eating protein directly supports muscle growth. Make sure you are eating at least 1.2 grams of protein per kilogram of body weight. For example, if you are 150 pounds, that translates to about 82 grams of protein per day, or 27 grams at each meal. For the average person, this likely means eating eggs or cottage cheese at breakfast and cheese, meat, or beans at lunch and dinner.

And hydrate! Every day, make sure you are taking in eight glasses of water. See chapter 14 for more on nutrition.

(☾) SLEEP

If you don't already sleep 7 to 8 hours a night, make a plan to start soon. You are training. You need rest to improve your fitness. See chapter 13 for more on sleep.

21 DAYS UNTIL TREATMENT

T minus 21 days until treatment

Today you will just do the five core lift movements 6 times. Then rest, and do the movements 6 more times. This is shown in the table at the end of the chapter as 2 sets of 6 reps. Light or no weight or resistance today—let's see how you feel tomorrow.

T minus 20 days until treatment

Day off from lifting. Notice whether and how much your body feels sore from yesterday's exercises. Don't forget that you still do the log, move, eat, and sleep components of the program even on days that you have off from lift.

T minus 19 days until treatment

You will be doing the five core lift exercises. Today you are doing more reps: 8 times, then resting, and then doing them again 8 times (2 sets of 8). Use enough resistance to make 2 sets of 8 challenging but not overwhelmingly difficult. Use your best judgment—you are allowed to change the weight based on how each set feels. If you are new to resistance exercise, start with the lightest weights you have. If the exercises feel too easy and you do not get sore the next day, increase the weight for the next session. If you are still sore from your last session, it is fine to do another session with no resistance. You should also do the log, move, eat, and sleep components today.

T minus 18 days until treatment

Day off from lifting. Notice whether and how much your body feels sore from yesterday's exercises. Be sure to do the log, move, eat, and sleep components today.

T minus 17 days until treatment

Today you are doing the five core lift movements 10 times each, for 2 sets (a total of 20 times for each movement). Use the same weights as the last session unless you are not getting sore at all from the prior sessions. If you are new to resistance exercise and you've started with 3- to 5-pound weights, you might find you can increase the resistance more quickly (and you might not). Also complete the log, move, eat, and sleep components today.

T minus 16 days until treatment

Day off from lifting. Notice whether and how much your body feels sore from yesterday's exercises. Also complete the log, move, eat, and sleep components today.

T minus 15 days until treatment

Today you are doing the five core lift movements 6 times each, for 3 sets (a total of 18 times for each movement). Use the same resistance as the last lift session—you are doing more work (more sets). Also complete the log, move, eat, and sleep components today.

T minus 14 days until treatment

Day off from lifting today. Notice whether the lift exercises are still leaving you sore, or whether your body is recovering more quickly from your weight-training sessions. Also complete the log, move, eat, and sleep components today.

T minus 13 days until treatment

Today you are again doing the five core lift movements 6 times, for 3 sets (a total of 18 times for each movement). Increase the resistance by no more than about 10 percent for each exercise. Sometimes that is not possible, so in those cases increase the weight by the smallest amount possible, getting as close to 10 percent as you can. For example, if you were using 10-pound dumbbells for an exercise, you should try to find 12-pound dumbbells for that exercise today. We know this is a 20 percent increase, but it's hard to find 11-pound dumbbells, so this is as close to 10 percent as you will likely get. In general, the resistance used for your lower body (squats, lunges, and deadlifts) should be higher than what you can do with your upper body (chest press and one-arm row).

When done correctly, you should really be working hard to finish the last few repetitions of each exercise in the last set. If you are not, increase the resistance more. Also complete the log, move, eat, and sleep components today.

T minus 12 days until treatment
Day off from lifting. Notice whether and how much your body feels sore from yesterday's increase in weight. Also complete the log, move, eat, and sleep components today.

T minus 11 days until treatment
Today you will be doing the five core lift movements 8 times each, for 3 sets (a total of 24 times for each movement). Use the same resistance you used for "T minus 13 days," unless it was too easy or too hard. Adjust as needed. Also complete the log, move, eat, and sleep components today.

T minus 10 days until treatment
Day off from lifting. Notice whether and how much your body is sore from yesterday's exercises. Also complete the log, move, eat, and sleep components today.

T minus 9 days until treatment
Continue progressing by doing the five lift movements 10 times, for 3 sets (a total of 30 times for each movement). Use the same resistance you used on "T minus 11 days," unless it was too easy or too hard. Adjust as needed. Also complete the log, move, eat, and sleep components today.

T minus 8 days until treatment
Day off from lifting. Notice whether and how much your body feels sore from yesterday's exercises. If you are still feeling sore the day after lifting,

try some recovery techniques like an Epsom salt bath or self-massage. Also complete the log, move, eat, and sleep components today.

T minus 7 days until treatment

Today you will be doing the five lift movements 6 times, for 4 sets each (a total of 24 times for each movement). Use the same resistance used on "T minus 9 days." Also complete the log, move, eat, and sleep components today.

T minus 6 days until treatment

Day off from lifting. As you complete the log, move, eat, and sleep components today, add an element that allows you to be mindful of how well you are doing in getting ready for the challenge to come. This can be as simple as a moment of reflection or a series of mindful breaths.

T minus 5 days until treatment

Today you are again doing the five lift movements 6 times, for 4 sets each (a total of 24 times for each movement); however, increase the resistance by 10 percent or so over the "T minus 7 days" level. For example, if you previously lifted 10 pounds, move up to 12 pounds. We know this is a 20 percent increase, but it's hard to find 11-pound dumbbells, so this is as close to 10 percent as you will likely get. Also complete the log, move, eat, and sleep components today.

T minus 4 days until treatment

Day off from lifting. By now doing the log, move, eat, and sleep components should be routine for you.

T minus 3 days until treatment

Today you are doing the five lift movements 8 times, for 4 sets (a total of 32 times for each movement). Use the same resistance as "T minus 5 days" unless it was too easy or too hard. Adjust as needed. Recall you should really have to work hard to complete the fourth set. You may not get all 8 repetitions completed if you are using the correct level of resistance. Also complete the log, move, eat, and sleep components today.

T minus 2 days until treatment

Day off from lifting. Log, move, eat, and sleep like a champ today.

T minus 1 day until treatment

Today you are doing the five lift movements 10 times, for 4 sets (a total of 40 times for each movement). Use the same resistance as "T minus 3 days," unless it was too easy or hard. Adjust as needed. Log, move, and eat in ways that allow you to feel you have mastered prehabilitation and make you proud of your preparation for treatment.

Sleep this night is what it is. Do your best and do not tell yourself you've done it wrong if you can't sleep the night before you begin treatment. Tomorrow's a big day, so give yourself a break!

Here's a chart of the program:

DAY T MINUS	MOVE	LIFT SETS	REPS	RESISTANCE	EAT	SLEEP
21	20–30 minutes	2	6	Zero	Eat 1.2 g of protein per kg of body weight and hydrate	Prioritize getting 8 hours a night
20	20–30 minutes			Off		
19	20–30 minutes	2	8	Make 2 sets of 8 reps hard but doable (guess, and then revise until you get it right)		
18	20–30 minutes			Off		
17	20–30 minutes	2	10	Same as day 19		

DAY T MINUS	MOVE	SETS	REPS	LIFT RESISTANCE	EAT	SLEEP
16	20–30 minutes			Off		
15	20–30 minutes	3	6	Same as day 19		
14	20–30 minutes			Off		
13	20–30 minutes	3	6	Increase by no more than 10%		
12	20–30 minutes			Off		
11	20–30 minutes	3	8	Same as day 13		
10	20–30 minutes			Off		
9	20–30 minutes	3	10	Same as day 13		
8	20–30 minutes			Off		
7	20–30 minutes	4	6	Same as day 13		
6	20–30 minutes			Off		
5	20–30 minutes	4	6	Increase by no more than 10%		
4	20–30 minutes			Off		
3	20–30 minutes	4	8	Same as day 5		
2	20–30 minutes			Off		
1	20–30 minutes	4	10	Same as day 5		
				Treatment starts		

SURGERY

There may be no cancer survivor in the world who understands recovering after surgery better than Dr. Susan Helmrich.

In 1977, at the age of twenty-one, she found out that she had two aggressive vaginal tumors. They were caused by the drug diethylstilbestrol, an FDA-approved medication her mother took during pregnancy that doctors subsequently learned increased a woman's risk for cancer of the cervix and vagina by about forty times. The ten-hour surgery to remove the tumors required a monthlong recovery in the hospital. At the time of her diagnosis, Helmrich had been an elite college swimmer; after her grueling recovery post-surgery, she found herself twenty-two years old and addicted to the opioids she was being prescribed for pain. "One day I realized, 'I don't think this is the life I want to live,'" she told me. Helmrich decided to go to her local YMCA and get back in the pool.

Fast-forward twenty years: Helmrich was now forty-one years old with children in first and third grade. Despite never having smoked a day in her life, she was diagnosed with a second cancer in her lung. Her surgeon took pains to salvage as much lung tissue as possible, yet Helmrich lost most of one of her lungs in the resulting operation. In the weeks after the surgery, she could barely walk around the block without gasping for air. Nevertheless, she knew from previous experience that moving and exercising as soon as possible would be good for her. She got back into the pool to swim and eventually race, despite the loss of nearly an entire lung.

Then twelve years later, at age fifty-three, the unthinkable occurred: Helmrich was diagnosed with a third tumor, this time in her pancreas. She underwent an operation known as a Whipple procedure to remove the tumor, an operation considered to be among the most major cancer surgeries performed.

All told, Helmrich has had eight cancer surgeries; she has had her left lung, gallbladder, duodenum, part of her pancreas, and all of her reproductive organs removed. And yet through all of it, Helmrich has continued swimming. At sixty-five, she remains a US Masters-level swimmer, having recently placed second in the 1650-meter freestyle and third in the 500-meter freestyle.

"I will be honest," Helmrich told me, "there's a lot of darkness. I was dealt the cards of a terrible body. There's so much wrong with my body—I've had a third of my organs removed. I have edema, I have sciatica, and there are so many foods that I can never eat again."

And yet swimming has been her lifeline. "Without swimming, I don't think I would have survived," she went on. "I started with one lap, then two laps, and every day I increased a little bit. What is the alternative—to sit in my room and crawl up in a ball and say, 'Oh, woe is me. I have cancer'?"

No one reading this book will have Helmrich's experience; it is unheard of to have three separate, seemingly unrelated cancer diagnoses in a lifetime. Her experience is one of a kind.

And yet it helps illustrate the extreme range of experiences cancer patients have with surgery. Surgery for cancer ranges from the minimally invasive skin cancer removal, where you walk out of the clinic the same day, to some of the most extensive and difficult procedures done in all of surgery, frequently requiring months of recovery.

The experience is also radically different depending on when and why you undergo surgery: You might be having surgery immediately after your diagnosis in order to retrieve a tissue sample of your tumor for testing, known as a biopsy; you may be undergoing surgery to remove your tumor entirely with the hope of a cure; or, finally, you may have surgery to help with the side effects of very advanced cancer, known as palliative surgery, even though there is no chance of a cure.

Helmrich's experience is also important because over the course of a life that includes eight cancer-related surgeries, she learned how to best recover from these operations. At twenty-two years old, not knowing any better, she relied too much on the painkillers she was prescribed. Twenty years later, having learned from her first experience, she began exercising as soon as she could after surgery. And after her most recent cancer surgery, the Whipple procedure, she asked for an exercise hand wheel in the hospital room so that she could begin moving as soon as possible. When she was able to walk, she did laps around the hospital floor pulling her IV pole.

It is interesting to note, however, that the advice she received from her doctors during this time did not change. "There was zero mention of exercise for my recovery," she said of her first operation in 1977. "Absolutely zero. I had no exercise advice. I was told to just go home and take as much Percocet as I wanted."

Four decades later, when she underwent her last major surgery, nothing had changed in her personal experience. "Again, no mention of exercise and no mention of nutrition."

But the wisdom of Helmrich's approach—to move early and often after surgery—has been borne out in dozens of studies, even though these recommendations are not always mentioned in surgery recovery rooms.

The best approach—and the one this book relies upon—is called "enhanced recovery after surgery," or ERAS for short. It is a collection of the best and most widely used techniques to "fast track" recovery from surgery. There are several steps in these "fast track" programs, some of which actually start before surgery, but in terms of exercise, the most important principle is this: early mobilization. Push yourself to move as early after surgery as possible and move as much as you safely and comfortably can. This cannot be overemphasized—move early and often after your surgery.

Many studies have shown that moving as soon as possible after surgery decreases the amount of time patients need to stay in the hospital; decreases the number and severity of unintended negative effects of surgery, or complications; and even decreases a person's chances of dying as a result of surgery.

These are very serious side effects of surgery. But moving early and often after surgery also helps in a bunch of small ways too. It will get your gut moving again. It will prevent your lungs from declining during the days of rest after surgery. It improves muscle function and physical strength and helps preserve the lean body mass you developed with your hard work training before surgery (see chapter 5). It is linked to getting back to your normal daily life more quickly after surgery and reducing fatigue, daytime sleep, and the number of sick days you need to use from work after surgery.

It is particularly important because the body's tissues decline and waste away shockingly fast when you're completely sedentary, as you may be after a cancer surgery. In the days and weeks of rest after surgery, you lose red blood cells, capillaries, and the infrastructure to deliver oxygen from your lungs to your tissues. You also lose muscle fiber as well as connective tissue, which binds bones and other tissue to each other.

In humans, some of the best evidence of the deleterious effects of bed rest we have comes from astronauts in space. On Earth, we are constantly fighting gravity; in fact, many of the resistance exercises throughout this book use nothing more than lifting your own body weight against the pull of gravity. But in zero-gravity conditions in space, daily physical work like moving around and lifting objects is not demanding. As a result, astronauts can lose up to 20 percent of their muscle mass on spaceflights that last between just five and eleven days. Dr. Jessica Scott, a researcher at Memorial Sloan Kettering Cancer Center, sees parallels between the experience of astronauts and cancer patients. The multiple system toxicities that occur in both space flight and cancer include cardiac atrophy, anemia, gastrointestinal events, exercise intolerance, muscle atrophy, and bone demineralization. Similar results have been found when medical researchers study the effects of long-term bedrest and immobilization, whether from surgery, diseases such as heart failure and diabetes, or neurodegenerative conditions such as Parkinson's and Huntington's or genetic muscle diseases. Put very simply, with muscle tissue in the human body, if you don't use it, you lose it. The good news is that even 10 minutes of simple movements a day can help prevent and reverse these problems.

THE PROGRAM:
TRAINING POST-SURGERY

The major difference in the program for this period of your treatment—the weeks post-surgery—is that there will be no lifting until your wounds have healed and your surgeon gives the all clear. The focus will be on the log, move, eat, and sleep aspects of the program.

 LOG

As with the pretreatment time frame, it will be useful for you to log symptoms, as well as your move, eat, and sleep habits, as you recover from surgery. The information could be helpful to your doctors to know how best to help you, and will prove to you what we already know: When you move, you feel better. Let those caring for you help with creating and filling out the daily log.

 MOVE

BEFORE YOU BEGIN
Recovering from cancer surgery has much less to do with your cancer than with the fact that you had surgery. Please consider your history of exercise before you start. For example, if you were running for 30-minute bouts prior to surgery, after you've been discharged from the hospital your exercise goal might be walking for 15 minutes. If you were sedentary and didn't regularly exercise prior to surgery, a good goal might be a 5-minute walk. Again, they are both incredibly helpful—the idea is simply to get moving quickly, but safely, as soon as possible after surgery. Your goal is to write down how much time you've moved daily and increase it a little bit every day, barring symptoms that you need

to back off (wound not healing, fever). Your goal is to get to 30 to 60 minutes a day.

Athletes are the most at risk of overdoing it after surgery. Your "muscle memory"—the neuromuscular connections that allow your brain to tell your muscles to move—is still intact and well-functioning after surgery. This means that you might be able to accomplish a big effort in the days after surgery, but you also risk injuring yourself or delaying your healing by, for example, pulling open your surgery wound or developing a hernia in the case of abdominal surgery. Over the long run, this will set you back significantly. Start slowly, listen to your body, and gradually progress. Be sure to follow the directions of your care team.

A fever is the clearest indication that something is going wrong after surgery. Pay attention to your temperature in the weeks post-surgery. Also, your wound should bleed less and look better as time passes, and pain should lessen as well. If any of these get worse, regardless of exercise, call your medical team.

If you are taking pain medication that makes you unsteady on your feet, hold on to the wall or a friend or relative when walking. The hope is that your need for the pain medication will decrease over time. If you have an active infection with a fever, do not exercise.

If wound healing, bleeding, or pain worsens during or after exercise, stop and try again the next day.

FIRST MOVEMENTS

Healing from your surgery is a form of physical work that must be honored. The time it takes to return to more than light activities will vary depending on the extent of your surgery. For example, if you had a small incision to remove something just under the skin, it may be as short as two weeks. On the other hand, if you had major abdominal surgery, it may take two months.

The goal during this period is to keep moving, mostly through walking or chair exercises. Start slowly and gradually build up. Begin with ankle pumping (pointing and flexing the toes) or ankle circles while you are still unable to get out of bed, just to get the circulation moving.

As soon as you are allowed after your surgery, start walking with your IV pole around the hospital floor, or even in your hospital room. March in place or step side to side if that's all the space you have available. Ask to have your athletic footwear brought to the hospital. Even if your first attempt results in 1 minute of movement, it's worth it. The next day you might be able to do 2 minutes. How many athletes can double their capacity in a day? You are a rock star!

Start with a few minutes a day and try to increase to 10 minutes a day during your hospital stay.

During the two to eight weeks immediately after surgery, when you are home, your focus should be on building *time* in aerobic activity, as opposed to building intensity. Increase your aerobic activity (walking or chair exercises) gradually to the point that you are doing between 150 and 300 minutes per week of moderate-intensity activity.

Wear well-fitting athletic shoes during your walks. In addition, stay hydrated by drinking a glass of water with every exercise session. If you are walking outside, be sure to protect yourself from the sun. If you find you are hungry after an exercise session, try to stick to fruits and vegetables. We don't burn that many calories per minute by walking, so don't make the mistake of thinking you've "earned" a candy bar. The average person will burn the equivalent of one cookie in a 30-minute walk (90 to 200 calories, depending on the person).

If you are eager to do more, remember that your body is working very hard to heal from the surgery and needs to spend energy on that, so you are already doing plenty. If you overdo it now at the beginning, you are lengthening the time it will take to heal completely. That's kind of like two steps forward, two steps back. Be patient.

If you don't feel like moving, remember that walking will likely make you feel better. Try for a few minutes and if you don't feel better, you can stop and try again the next day.

If there are other exercises your medical team has prescribed (such as breathing or Kegel exercises), please do them regularly. Studies show that those who perform these types of exercises recover better and faster. Consider asking for a referral to physical therapy if it is not automatically offered so that you enjoy the full expertise from these important professionals.

CHAIR EXERCISE ROUTINE

A YouTube-style video of this exercise program is available at www.movingthroughcancer.com.

If you or your care team think it is inadvisable for you to walk, try this chair exercise routine. It should take about 10 minutes to complete the whole thing. Build up to 1 complete set (10 minutes a day), then progress to 2 sets (20 minutes a day) in a session, then finally 3 sets (30 minutes a day). If any of these cause pain near your incision, skip that one and move on to the next one.

··

CHAIR MARCHES

March in place in the chair for 1 minute.

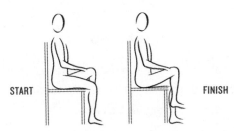

START   FINISH

QUARTER TURNS

Open the right leg by stepping the right foot out to the right side, move the left leg to match it, then return to center; open the left leg by stepping the left foot out to the left side, move the right leg to match it, then return to center. Repeat for 1 minute.

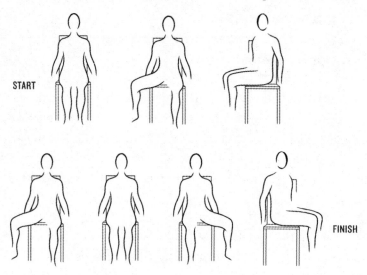

LEANING

Reach the fingers of the right hand toward the ground, then sit up straight; reach the fingers of the left hand toward the ground, then sit up straight. Repeat for 1 minute.

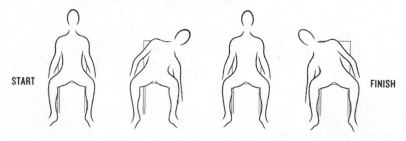

STAND AND SIT

Stand up from the chair and sit down. Repeat for 1 minute.

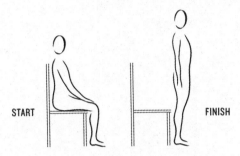

START

FINISH

LEG EXTENSIONS

Sit up straight and extend the right leg to horizontal (parallel to the ground), toes pointed to the ceiling. Return to the starting position, then repeat with the left leg. Repeat for 1 minute.

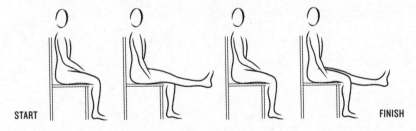

START

FINISH

STAR

Extend the arms and legs out at the same time, like a star shape, then return the legs and arms to the starting position. Repeat for 1 minute.

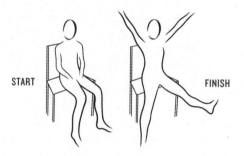

OPPOSING ARM AND LEG WINDMILLS

Reach the right arm to the left ankle, left arm behind; return to center and repeat on the other side. Repeat for 1 minute.

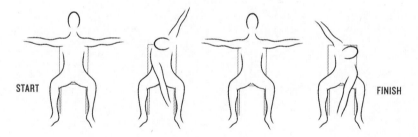

FORWARD BENDS

With arms resting on the lap, lean forward toward the knees, allowing arms to reach toward toes. Hold for 2 seconds; return to seated. Repeat for 1 minute.

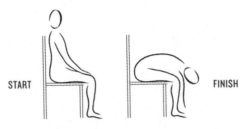

START   FINISH

TURNING AROUND

Turn the head and shoulders to the left, place the left elbow on the chair back, and reach around to your left side with your right arm. Leave the knees facing front. Repeat on the other side. Repeat for 1 minute.

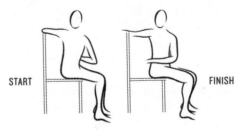

START   FINISH

CALF RAISES

Can be done seated or standing behind the chair, holding on to the back of the chair. Rise up on the balls of the feet and lower back down. Repeat for 1 minute.

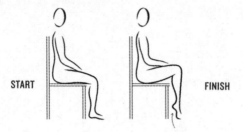

START   FINISH

EXERCISES FOR SPECIFIC SURGERIES

HEAD AND NECK SURGERIES
(cancers of the head and neck, brain tumors, and skin cancers)
Focus on: Building *time* in aerobic activity, as opposed to building intensity. Increase your aerobic activity (mostly walking during this period) gradually to the point that you are doing between 150 and 300 minutes per week of moderate-intensity activity. Do not restart any resistance exercise activities until your stitches have been removed and your wounds are fully closed. The length of time this takes varies from person to person and according to the size of the wound being healed. Your surgeon will help you decide when you are able to return to resistance exercise. In addition, given where you've had your surgery, it's not a time to do activities that require your head to be lower than your heart, which is the case in many stretching and yoga activities.

BREAST CANCER SURGERY
Focus on: Building *time* in aerobic activity, as opposed to building intensity. Increase your aerobic activity (mostly walking during this period) gradually to the point that you are doing between 150 and 300 minutes per week of moderate-intensity activity. The weeks after breast cancer surgery are not a time for resistance exercise. In addition, given where you've had your surgery, it's important that you not overstretch or strain your chest, shoulders, or upper back. Work with a physical therapist before choosing to restart any resistance exercise activities while you still have drains and stitches and until your wounds are fully closed. The number of weeks this takes will vary from person to person and according to the type of surgery. Women who undergo a lumpectomy with no reconstruction will generally recover much faster than women who undergo a full mastectomy with reconstruction. Your surgeon will help you decide when you are able to return to resistance exercise. To ensure that you maintain a full range of motion in your shoulders after breast or thoracic cancer surgeries, do the "wall crawl" exercise shown on the next page.

THORACIC SURGERIES
(cancers in the lungs, esophagus, trachea, heart, or diaphragm)

Focus on: Building *time* in aerobic activity, as opposed to building intensity. Increase your aerobic activity (should be mostly walking at this time) gradually to the point that you are doing between 150 and 300 minutes per week of moderate-intensity activity. Follow the walking recommendations at the start of this section to avoid surgical complications. Avoid straining for any reason until the surgical wound has healed.

To ensure that you maintain a full range of motion in your shoulders after breast or thoracic cancer surgeries, do the following "wall crawl" exercise:

....

WALL CRAWLS

Stand facing the wall and crawl the fingers of one hand up until the hand is extending straight up, then walk toward the wall until you feel a stretch in the arm and shoulder. Repeat 10 times, rest, and perform another set of 10. Do the exercise on both sides, in part so that you can see how the unaffected side moves and know what is possible for the affected side once you've fully healed.

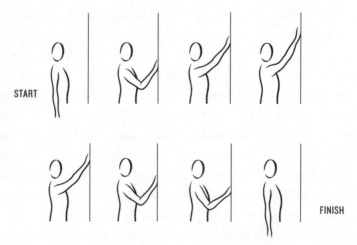

ABDOMINAL SURGERIES
(colorectal cancer and many gastrointestinal cancers affecting the stomach and digestive system)

Focus on: Healing. Keep moving, but heal. It is really important for your recovery that you follow the walking recommendations at the start of this section to avoid surgical complications. During this period your focus should be on building *time* in aerobic activity, as opposed to building intensity. Increase your aerobic activity (should be mostly walking at this time) gradually to the point that you are doing between 150 and 300 minutes per week of moderate-intensity activity.

To avoid the risk of an incisional hernia, follow your doctor's advice as to when you can return to resistance exercise. Most people can return to all activities within six to eight weeks. That said, abdominal surgeries weaken the core muscles, so it is important that you begin the process of restrengthening them as soon as it is safe to do so. Here are a few simple and safe things that can be started in the weeks after surgery.

....

HEAD LIFTS WHILE LYING ON THE BED

Lie on your back with your knees bent. Lift your head off the bed and hold for a few seconds, then rest your head down. Try 10, rest, repeat.

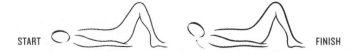

START   FINISH

BUTT LIFTS/BRIDGES

Lie on your back, on the floor or on your bed, with your knees bent. Lift the buttocks and hold for a few seconds, then release back to the floor/bed. Try 10, rest, repeat.

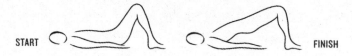

START · · · · · · · · · · · · · · · · · · FINISH

KNEE TWISTS

Lie down with your knees bent and feet flat on the floor. From this starting position, allow your knees to drop to the right side, and stretch your arms out into a "T" position. Return your knees to center. Drop your knees to the left side and stretch your arms out into a "T" position. Return your knees to the center again. Repeat 10 per side, rest, and repeat.

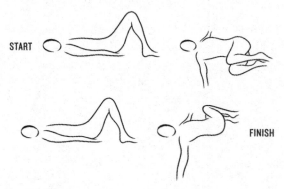

START

FINISH

PELVIC SURGERIES
(cancers of the prostate and female reproductive organs)

Focus on: Kegel exercises (see opposite page) to strengthen the pelvic floor as soon as your surgical team allows you to start. Beyond that, the general instructions for ankle circles, walking with the IV pole, and increasing walking to between 150 and 300 minutes per week should be followed to ensure the best possible recovery.

Kegel exercises are intended to strengthen the muscles of the pelvic floor. It is advisable that you ask for a referral to a physical therapist after pelvic surgery so that you can be instructed in person how to do these exercises most effectively. Until that is possible, the basic instructions are included in the figure below.

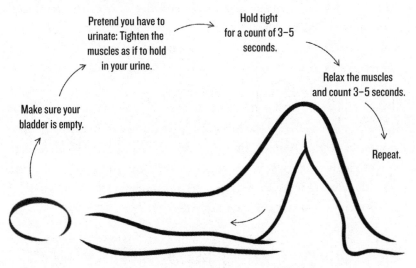

Pretend you have to urinate: Tighten the muscles as if to hold in your urine.

Hold tight for a count of 3–5 seconds.

Relax the muscles and count 3–5 seconds.

Make sure your bladder is empty.

Repeat.

EXTREMITY SURGERIES
(sarcomas and skin cancers resulting in surgeries to the arms, hands, legs, and feet)

Focus on: The walking recommendations at the start of this section to avoid surgical complications. During this period your focus should be on building *time* in aerobic activity, as opposed to building intensity. Increase your aerobic activity (should be mostly walking at this time) gradually to the point that you are doing between 150 and 300 minutes per week of moderate-intensity activity.

There is a concentrated program of functional recovery for those who undergo limb amputation. Follow the directions of your physical therapist to ensure the best and fastest possible return to as much function as possible.

⊗ EAT

If there are aspects of nutrition that are emphasized for surgical recovery, they tend to focus on whole foods, fiber, protein, and foods that boost the immune system. Eating whole foods refers to eating a food as it is in nature, rather than how it might be processed into something else. An example would be to eat an apple rather than an apple pie. Fiber is useful after surgery because of the common experience of constipation during recovery from anesthesia. Increasing fiber in your diet could help with avoiding or improving constipation. Protein intake should be high while you recover from surgery. Try to eat protein with every meal. Your body is rebuilding and repairing tissue and that takes a lot of protein. Finally, there are some foods that are thought to boost immune function. Given the risk for infection and the focus on the immune system helping repair body tissues after a surgery, consider adding citrus fruits, red bell peppers, broccoli, garlic, ginger, spinach, yogurt (Greek yogurt is high in protein), almonds, sunflower seeds, turmeric, green tea, papaya, and kiwi to your diet. See chapter 14 for more on nutrition.

☾ SLEEP

Rest is a key element in recovery from surgery. As noted above, it takes energy to heal, and you need your rest to have sufficient energy for healing. Sleep disturbances after surgery can slow your recovery. One of the key issues that gets in the way of sleep post-surgery is symptom management. There are both medication and non-medication approaches to improving your sleep after surgery. Avoid opioid-containing medications, which have been shown to disturb sleep, even when they effectively treat pain. Sleep medications that are effective for post-surgery patients include zolpidem, melatonin, and dexmedetomidine.

Non-drug approaches relate to the "sleep hygiene" approaches commonly used for improving sleep in the general population. In short, sleep hygiene refers to carrying out a number of steps to improve your sleep, such as avoiding caffeine, exercising regularly, eliminating noise and light from the sleeping area, and maintaining a regular sleep schedule. For post-surgical patients, perhaps one aspect that would be worth logging is the effect of naps on nighttime sleep. If you log naps and note that you don't sleep well on a day when you nap longer than 30 minutes, set an alarm to end your naps in 30 minutes. Your goal is to get 7 to 8 hours of sleep per night. See chapter 13 for more on sleep.

Here is a chart of the program for three weeks after surgery:

DAY SINCE SURGERY	MOVE	SPECIAL EXERCISES SPECIFIC TO SURGERY TYPE	EAT	SLEEP
1	Get out of bed if possible	Do the special exercises as described earlier in the chapter (e.g., Kegels for pelvic surgery, core exercises for abdominal surgery, wall crawls for thoracic and breast surgery) as well as any exercises prescribed by your care team. Adhering to these predicts good outcomes!	Whole foods, fiber, protein, and immune-boosting foods (such as citrus fruits, red bell peppers, broccoli, garlic, ginger, spinach, yogurt, almonds, sunflower seeds, turmeric, green tea, papaya, and kiwi). See chapter 14 for more on nutrition.	Prioritize 8 hours a night, follow sleep hygiene guidance, and limit naps to 30 minutes or less. See chapter 13 for more on sleep.
2	Increase time out of bed by 2–3 minutes			
3	Increase time out of bed by 2–3 minutes			
4	Increase time out of bed by 2–3 minutes			
5	1 round of chair exercise routine			
6	2 rounds of chair exercise routine			
7	3 rounds of chair exercise routine or walk 10–30 minutes, as you are able; feel free to break up the movement into several sessions (e.g., 10 minutes in the morning, 10 minutes in the evening)			
8–21	Continue to gradually increase walking or chair exercise rounds until you can do 30–60 minutes per day			

WORKING WITH YOUR CARE TEAM

For some, surgery will be the most debilitating single experience of cancer treatment. If you are worried about whether it is OK for you to do the exercises outlined in this chapter, please see a physical therapist. Take this chapter directly to them and ask, "Do you have any concerns or questions? Is there anything you think I shouldn't do?" They may provide some guidance based on your unique medical history. Ask for a referral to physical therapy from your surgeon or oncologist—if you have cancer and your doctor makes a referral to physical therapy, the visit should be paid for by insurance.

Finally, there may be a long delay between your surgery and your next treatment, perhaps as long as six months in some cases. If you've completed the surgery recovery program outlined in this chapter and are still in between treatments, go back and do the prehabilitation program in chapter 5. This will maintain your fitness and prepare your body for the next treatment to come.

CHEMO
AND OTHER INFUSION THERAPIES

t is one of the most common misconceptions we hear from those undergoing chemotherapy treatments: Surely chemo, with its difficult infusion treatments and awful side effects, means that I should stop exercising and save my strength, right?

"My patients always ask me that—should I stop exercising when I'm getting chemo?" my friend and colleague, oncologist Dr. Natalie Marshall, told me when I asked her about this. "And I say, 'Absolutely not. You should continue exercising. And you should even increase your exercise.'"

Dr. Marshall treats breast and lung cancer patients in Berkeley, California, where she directs the University of California San Francisco-John Muir Health Cancer Center. She's been recommending exercise to her cancer patients for two decades based on the latest evidence in the field.

"I really encourage people to do strength training. I try to get them walking first and then as soon as they are getting to where they can walk more, I add strength training. Strength training is key because they need to actually build muscle mass and change the fat-mass-to-muscle-mass ratio in order to have the very best benefit."

WHY DO WE USE DRUGS THAT ARE SO TOXIC TO TREAT CANCER?

All of the drugs used to treat cancer are designed to keep cancer cells from multiplying. These treatments are systemic, meaning they travel throughout the entire body. This allows them to attack both the original, primary tumor as well as any cancer cells that have traveled, or metastasized, to other parts of the body.

However, it also means that cancer drugs may damage healthy but rapidly multiplying cells in the body. For example, chemotherapy may kill blood-forming cells in the bone marrow, hair follicles, and cells in the mouth, digestive tract, and reproductive system. Cancer treatments are often toxic to these cells, and the damage it causes are the drug's side effects.

COMMON DRUG THERAPIES FOR CANCER

The most common, and well-known, systemic treatment for cancer is *chemotherapy*. Cancer cells tend to form new cells more quickly than normal cells. Though specific chemotherapies work in different ways, they all keep cancer cells from reproducing. Doctors give chemo in cycles, with each period of treatment followed by a rest period to give you time to recover from the effects of the drugs. The length of cycle varies depending on the kind of cancer, and the schedule of drug delivery varies depending on the regimen used.

Sometimes a cancer cell replicates more quickly because of a mutated gene that occurs only in the cancer cells, not in normal tissue. A *targeted therapy* will home in on specific proteins or enzymes linked to that mutated gene, disrupting the growth of new cancer cells.

Certain cancers that affect the sex organs, such as breast, ovarian, or prostate cancer, may depend on hormones to grow. *Hormone therapy* stops or slows the growth of these kinds of cancer by preventing the body from making a specific hormone, blocking the hormone from attaching to cancer cells, or altering the hormone so it does not work like it should. We will discuss hormone therapy more specifically in chapter 9.

Immunotherapy is one of the newest forms of cancer treatment. It uses the body's own immune system to fight cancer. Though there are many different kinds of immunotherapies, most work by activating the immune system to find and kill cancer cells.

Infusion Therapies and Side Effects

Each of these regimens, treatments, and individual drugs has its own set of side effects and timing during which symptoms are most severe. One of the most important points to understand, and often the most confusing as well, is that these side effects will feel different—sometimes slightly different, sometimes incredibly different—each day during the course of treatment.

Let's use the most common side effect, fatigue, as an example. Patients undergoing chemotherapy often feel the most fatigued in the days right after treatment. It is typically most severe several days after treatment, after which energy gradually starts to increase. In one study of twenty-seven breast cancer patients, side effects such as fatigue peaked between three and five days after the day of treatment and had largely subsided by the next treatment date. Side effects like fatigue tend to follow a pattern:

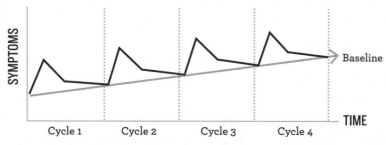

Pattern of symptoms over successive chemotherapy cycles

What you will note in the above figure is that while the symptoms did get better after the peak (during the recovery period), they did not come back down to the baseline level. That is because the effects of chemotherapy are cumulative, building up over successive cycles. Basically, this means that you feel a little bit worse with every cycle. So you will be able to do your best with exercise during cycle one of chemotherapy and what you will be able to accomplish may diminish as you progress through therapy. It's OK that you may do less as cycles go on. You will recover. The fact that you are doing something should be your focus.

The good news is that exercise has been shown to reduce chemotherapy side effects, which has important ramifications for finishing your prescribed course of treatment and achieving the best possible outcome.

BENEFITS OF EXERCISE

As we mentioned in earlier chapters, the 2019 American College of Sports Medicine Roundtable on Exercise for Cancer Prevention and Control concluded that there was sufficient scientific evidence that exercise during chemotherapy can improve cancer-related fatigue, as well as depression and anxiety. Sleep is also improved with exercise during chemotherapy. Further, exercise improves quality of life and physical function during chemotherapy. For these last two items, perhaps a translation is in order. What we mean by improved "quality of life" is the sense that life is worth living and has quality. "Physical function" refers to your ability to do all the things you are used to doing physically. There is published evidence that cancer patients have a decline in physical function over the period of treatment that is about equivalent to a decade of aging. One of my studies shows that exercise can prevent these declines in physical function from happening.

In addition, there is emerging evidence that exercise may have another important effect: It can help you complete treatment as prescribed by your doctor. This is important because finishing your full schedule of treatments directly affects your likelihood of reaching five years cancer free.

We've mentioned this research before, but it is so specifically relevant to chemotherapy, we are repeating this information for emphasis. There are two important medical studies that have looked at the effects of exercise on chemotherapy completion rate. They first looked at 242 women who were just about to start chemotherapy after having surgery to remove their breast cancers. The researchers randomly assigned them to one of three groups: The first was asked to do regular aerobic exercise; the second was asked to do a regular program of strength training and aerobic exercise; and the third was not asked to change their exercise habits at all.

After four months, the researchers doing the study found a few things they expected: Aerobic exercise helped preserve patients' fitness during the progressive cycles of chemotherapy and prevented them from adding any fat to their bodies (as much as 80 percent of women gain weight after a breast cancer diagnosis). Strength training improved muscular strength and preserved lean body mass. Both intervention types improved women's self-esteem, which is very important during the physically and emotionally draining experience of chemotherapy. But they also found something they didn't expect: The group that did strength training improved their ability to finish treatments as prescribed.

The cumulative side effects mentioned above are one of the main reasons patients don't make it all the way through treatment, in addition to some that count as medical emergencies, like the ability to fight off a serious infection. If you can get through the side effects that are not emergencies and receive more than 85 percent of your planned treatments, you are doing well. But below 85 percent, you may not be getting the maximum benefit from your treatments. As an example, between a quarter and a third of women with early breast cancer—the group of women included in the study above—do not ultimately reach 85 percent of their planned chemotherapy treatments.

Medical emergencies like a serious infection cannot always be prevented. But for the first time, the study showed something incredibly promising: that cancer patients could take action through a combined program of aerobic exercise and strength training to improve their chances of finishing chemotherapy.

A group of researchers in Amsterdam also looked at this question. In their study, 230 men and women with breast or colon cancer were again randomly assigned to one of three programs: a group that did at least 30 minutes of low-intensity physical activity five days a week; a group that did higher-intensity combined aerobic and strength-training sessions supervised by a specially trained physical therapist twice a week, plus additional lower-intensity exercising throughout the remainder of the week; and a group that did not change their activity level at all. Essentially, the researchers were trying to compare low-intensity exercise done in the home with combined aerobic and strength training done in supervised training sessions in a gym. These exercise programs were done for the entirety of the research participants' chemotherapy treatments.

This time the results were even more dramatic. Of the patients who did no exercise or the lower intensity walking-only program, 34 percent required a reduction in the amount of chemotherapy because of symptoms or infections. In contrast, only 12 percent of the patients who did higher intensity, combined aerobic and strength training needed to reduce their treatments. The researchers also found that the patients who did combined aerobic and strength training had better overall fitness and muscle strength and less fatigue than those in the other groups.

We specifically want to highlight that this research showed a particularly important role of strength training. Low-intensity exercise like regular walking was certainly helpful, but the real benefits came from adding strength training to the exercise mix and progressing the weights gradually but regularly. Exercise scientists believe that this benefit may come from preserving lean muscle mass, though we're still learning much more. This is why we include strength training in our recommended program that follows.

THE PROGRAM:
TRAINING DURING INFUSION THERAPY

We know how patients are likely to feel during chemotherapy. The exercise program we recommend is designed to make you feel better and tolerate your treatments better. We know that it is effective for a broad number of common symptoms that patients experience during chemotherapy. Further, doing what is recommended here could result in being able to complete your chemotherapy as originally prescribed, which may increase your chances of long-term survival.

We also know that during chemotherapy, patients report having "good days" and "bad days." The pattern of good and bad days will vary according to whether your chemotherapy regimen is delivered once every three weeks, once every two weeks, weekly, or daily in pill form. There are also the cognitive effects of chemotherapy. To quote one patient, "I couldn't remember the word 'potato' on bad days." As a result, we planned the program that follows to be really simple. Here are the rules:

Even on your bad days:

- Walk, ideally for 30 minutes. It's not good for anyone to sit on the sofa all day. The body is meant to be in motion. If you can call a friend to have a coffee, you can walk. If you can watch television, you can walk. Get your family, children, and friends to walk with you. If you don't have an obvious fitness buddy, contact 2unstoppable.org. They find fitness buddies for cancer patients and survivors. Earn the right to sit on that sofa the rest of the day.

On good days, the goal is to do:

- 30 minutes of aerobic activity that makes you breathe hard 3 times per week. This could simply mean walking faster than usual.

- Twice-weekly strength training (with one day between strength-training sessions).

You will know your bad days. Those are the days when you cannot concentrate enough to watch television and the days when you are mostly bedridden. If you can concentrate enough to watch TV, you can lift some weights or walk for at least 10 minutes.

📋 LOG

Your log becomes more important during chemotherapy. It will be your guide whether to walk or do something more.

First, you need to log your exercise, symptoms, sleep, and protein intake. As described in chapter 2, your support system can help with this. Perhaps there could be a star chart rather than a log. You could have some fun with this: Maybe you earn something after five days of exercise in a row?

Within the log, you will want to record your level of fatigue once a day, beginning on the day of your first infusion. Your doctor may want you to record other symptoms as well. This log can help you help your doctor in making sure you are safe and well during chemotherapy.

If fatigue and other symptoms are on the rise, you may choose to take a day off from lifting, as that would be a "peak symptom day," but you would still walk for 30 minutes. Even if you walk for 10 minutes and stop to throw up, walk. For most people, symptoms generally tend to be better in the hours and days after an exercise session. Pay close attention and find the patterns given your particular chemotherapy regimen. And if you feel well enough to exercise, get to it! Your symptoms might not allow for an exercise session tomorrow.

Use your log to organize your exercise sessions to avoid peak symptom days. Given that your goal is three move sessions and two lift sessions per week, that may mean doubling up on some days—doing aerobic exercise and strength training on the same day. This will be particularly true if your fatigue and other symptoms prevent you from exercising for more than two days in a given week.

That said, it is important never to lift two days in a row. The muscles require at least 48 hours to recover between sessions. If you are someone who is used to doing strength training, you might find you need more recovery time than usual during chemotherapy. You should at least *try* to do the prescribed exercises on the suggested schedule. You will know whether you need to stop.

(✗) MOVE

For the aerobic exercise sessions, the goal varies according to whether you are having a "bad day" versus a "good day." On a bad day, you walk, ideally for 30 minutes. That is your baseline. It is nonnegotiable. On good days, the goal is to do an activity that you enjoy, one that raises your heart rate enough so that you breathe heavier, and to maintain that activity for 30 minutes. As to how hard you should be working, we know that chemotherapy changes the way the heart rate responds to exercise. Because of this, it is important to use your perceived level of effort to discern how hard you are working, rather than your heart rate response. Recall from prior chapters that perceived effort uses a simple 1 to 10 scale, where 1 is sitting on the couch with the remote in hand and 10 is running as fast as you can, like to catch a bus or a plane. Aim for an intensity of 4 to 6 on this scale.

Another way to think of exercise intensity is using the "breath test." For light activities, you should be able to breathe through your nose only. Moderate activities are done at a "conversational pace"—you can talk in complete sentences but you cannot sing. At a vigorous level of activity, you have trouble talking and may be out of breath. You are aiming for that point between moderate and vigorous.

As to what kinds of activities are appropriate for aerobic exercise, here's a list of ideas for you:

- Walking faster than usual

- Jogging

- Cycling (outdoors or stationary)

- Dancing (just turn on some music and go!)

- Exercise DVDs

- Online exercise classes from trusted sources

- Gym classes such as Zumba or step aerobics

Some people prefer to do their exercise in the company of others, and that's fine. However, your immune system is not at its best during chemotherapy, so check with your medical team to see whether they are OK with you heading to the gym or to group fitness classes during treatment.

LIFT

For the strength program, your goal is to counteract the loss of muscle mass that we know occurs during chemotherapy. You will be performing the same five exercises from the prehabilitation program: chest press, one-arm row, squats, lunges, and deadlifts. You should be familiar with these movements from chapter 5, but we will show them and describe them for you again here as well. If you want more variety, go to my website, www.movingthroughcancer.com. The recommended exercises are as follows:

....

CHEST PRESS

Lie on your back on a weight-lifting bench, an aerobic step, or on the floor on a towel. Starting with arms straight, bend your elbows to right angles, elbows away from the body, then return arms to straight over your chest. When you add resistance, this will become challenging.

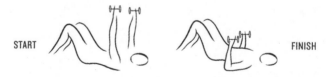

ONE-ARM ROW

Place one knee and one hand on a chair or the edge of the bed, as shown in the illustrations. Start with your free hand hanging down. Squeeze your shoulder blade toward your spine as you bend your elbow to raise your fist toward your side. Slowly lower to the starting position. Switch and do the other side.

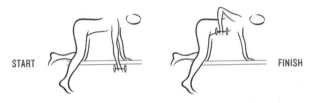

START   FINISH

SQUATS

Stand in front of a full-length mirror, facing to the side. Your feet should be hip distance apart, toes pointed forward. Hold your weights by your sides (like suitcases), as shown. Sit backward as if you are going to sit down in a chair, keeping your chest lifted, eyes forward. In fact, to start, keep a chair behind you, so that if you touch the chair, you will know you've gone down far enough. Sneak a peek at your knees in the mirror: They shouldn't bend past 90 degrees. Sneak a peek at your knees by looking down: Your knees should not go out past your toes and should stay parallel (not drift toward or away from each other).

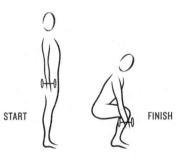

START   FINISH

LUNGES

Hold on to a chair or the wall and step backward with one foot so that you can bend both knees to 90-degree angles, while keeping your chest up. Return to the starting position. Repeat for a full set on one side before switching to the other leg. If you can do lunges without holding on, that's great too. To add resistance for the supported lunge, hold on with one hand and hold a weight in the other hand, at your side.

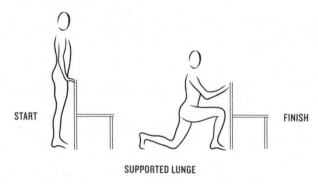

START   FINISH

SUPPORTED LUNGE

DEADLIFTS

Stand with your feet hip-width apart. Bend just at the hips, letting the head follow the back so you are looking at the floor at the end of the movement. Return to standing.

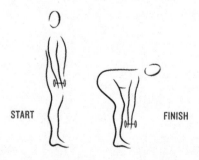

START   FINISH

Do each movement 10 times. Then rest for a minute, then do each movement 10 times again. In exercise parlance, that's 2 sets of 10 repetitions. As you feel able, increase the resistance. That may or may not be possible for you during chemotherapy. That's OK! When chemotherapy is over, you can work to get stronger. For now, it's a reasonable goal to maintain the strength you have.

This is far less resistance exercise than when you were in the prehabilitation phase, in acknowledgment of how hard it will be to do all this exercise during chemotherapy. What we recommend here is the scientifically proven dose of exercise to improve your symptoms.

⊗ EAT

During chemotherapy, it is particularly recommended that you take in adequate protein. Further guidance on eating throughout treatment can be found in chapter 14.

☾ SLEEP

Sleep can become disturbed during chemotherapy for a number of reasons, including because of long naps during the day. Try to keep your nap length under an hour to ensure that you get adequate nighttime sleep. Proper sleep hygiene approaches to help promote a good night's rest are outlined in chapter 13.

HOW IT ALL COMES TOGETHER

We recognize that chemotherapy is delivered on many schedules. Our goal is to make it simple to keep moving during chemotherapy. To make this all come together during chemotherapy requires a bit of organization. We recommend making a blank log like the one from chapter 2 or downloading it from my website, www.movingthroughcancer.com.

Here's an example of a good week:

		SUN	MON	TUE
	GOOD DAY / BAD DAY	Good	Good	Good
	FATIGUE 0 – 10 (10 = WORST)	5	6	4
	OTHER SYMPTOMS 0 – 10 (10 = WORST)	5 Nausea	3 Nausea	2 Nausea
	SLEEP 0 – 10 (10 = BEST)	7 woke twice 8 hours	7 woke 3 times 6 hours	7 woke twice 7 hours
	MOVE* ★ (PER 30 MIN)	★ Dancing, 30 minutes		★ Dancing, 30 minutes
	LIFT ★ (PER SESSION)		★ 5 exercises, 2x each	
	PROTEIN† # SERVINGS	4 Protein shake, chicken, eggs	2 Protein shake x2	4 Protein shake, burger, eggs

*Move goal varies according to where you are in treatment (less during chemotherapy and radiation). See chapters 5–11.

† See chapter 13 for guidance on how much protein you need. For the purposes of this chart, either add up the total grams of protein eaten each day or the number of servings: 1 serving = 3 oz of meat/poultry/fish, ½ cup cottage cheese or yogurt, 1 egg, 1 cup of milk, 1 cup of lentils/beans, or 1 protein drink/bar

WED	THU	FRI	SAT
Good	Good	Good	Good
3	3	3	3
0 No	0 No	0 No	0 No
7 woke twice 7 hours	7 woke 3 times 7 hours	9 woke once 7 hours	10 slept through 8 hours
	★ Brisk walk, 30 minutes		
★ 5 exercises, 2x each			
4 Eggs, protein shake x2	4 Eggs, protein shake x2	3 Chicken, protein shake x2	4 Eggs, protein shake x2

NOTES:

Sunday: felt better after dancing. Tuesday: felt better after dancing.

Thursday: feeling strong!

Here's an example of a really tough (but successful) week:

		SUN	MON	TUE
	GOOD DAY / BAD DAY	Bad	Bad	Bad
	FATIGUE 0 – 10 (10 = WORST)	7	8	9
	OTHER SYMPTOMS 0 – 10 (10 = WORST)	7 Nausea	7 Nausea	5 Nausea
	SLEEP 0 – 10 (10 = BEST)	5 tossed and turned	5 tossed and turned	6 tossed and turned
	MOVE* ★ (PER 30 MIN)	★ Walk, 30 minutes	★ Walk, 30 minutes	★ Walk, 30 minutes
	LIFT ★ (PER SESSION)	No	No	No
	PROTEIN† # SERVINGS	Everything tastes like chalk this week	½ Protein shake	1 Protein shake

*Move goal varies according to where you are in treatment (less during chemotherapy and radiation). See chapters 5–11.

† See chapter 13 for guidance on how much protein you need. For the purposes of this chart, either add up the total grams of protein eaten each day or the number of servings: 1 serving = 3 oz of meat/poultry/fish, ½ cup cottage cheese or yogurt, 1 egg, 1 cup of milk, 1 cup of lentils/beans, or 1 protein drink/bar

WED	THU	FRI	SAT
Bad	Bad	Bad	Bad
9	9	9	10
5 Nausea	Neuropathy 3 Nausea 5	Neuropathy 3 Nausea 3	Neuropathy 3 Nausea 7
5 tossed and turned	5 tossed and turned	5 tossed and turned	5 tossed and turned
★ Walk, 30 minutes	★ Walk, 30 minutes	★ Walk, 30 minutes	Day in bed
No	No	No	No
1 Protein shake	1 Protein shake	$^1/_2$ Protein shake	$^1/_2$ Protein shake

NOTES:

Sunday: I hate walking, but I feel better afterward. Tuesday: walking really does help. Wednesday: managed to walk 15 minutes in the morning and 15 in the afternoon. Friday: struggled to get the walking done today.

We recommend that your *baseline* be walking, ideally 30 minutes a day, during chemotherapy because this is what you can do to help your doctors treat your cancer. This is what is in *your* control. You do not benefit from sitting on the sofa for the whole day. Get a family member or friend to go with you and walk. Just walk. It's raining? Take an umbrella. If it makes you feel better to hate us while doing it, we are OK with that. That's how confident we are that this will help you.

TIMING AND ALTERNATIVE APPROACHES

You may find that your energy is higher during the earlier part of the day, so try getting your exercise done before lunch. Further, there is one alternative way to perform the strength-training program, even if your day is trending toward a bad one: Split up the exercises. You could choose to do the two exercises for the upper body (chest press and one-arm row) on one day and the three exercises for the lower body (squats, lunges, and deadlifts) the next day. If this makes it more likely that you will be able to complete the lift program, give it a try.

RADIATION

"**W**hen people think of cancer treatment, radiation is probably one of the last treatments they think about. And it's the one they know the least about. Most people, when they think of cancer treatment, think of either surgery or chemotherapy." That was my colleague Dr. Nick Zaorsky's response when I asked how his patients view his treatments. Dr. Zaorsky is a radiation oncologist at Penn State University, where he leads the prostate cancer radiation oncology program. He and I have launched a number of clinical trials together that study how exercise helps people who are receiving radiation for advanced cancer. We know it will improve the quality of their lives; we also think it will help them live longer, and that's what these studies are designed to test.

Dr. Zaorsky's sentiment rings true. For many people given a cancer diagnosis, radiation is the last thing on their mind. Yet half of people with cancer require radiation treatments, and the majority of them receive radiation with the goal that it will help cure them of their cancer. Outside of surgery, radiation is the most important treatment that medicine has to cure cancer.

So it follows that you want to be in the best shape you can to complete your treatments. And this is where we already know exercise can really help. The main benefit of moving as much as possible in between your radiation treatments, whether it's aerobic exercise or strength training, is that it will reduce your side effects. And in particular, exercise helps with the most widespread problem people feel during radiation—fatigue.

"I tell patients that unless they have some specific reason not to exercise or move around, they should be as active as they can be," Dr. Zaorsky told me. "You're not going to feel worse—you're going to feel better. You should be able to handle your cancer treatments better and the quality of your life should improve."

HOW RADIATION IS USED TO TREAT CANCER

Radiation treatments, which are sometimes called radiotherapy or simply radiation, use high-energy particles or waves, such as x-rays, gamma rays, electron beams, or protons, to destroy or damage cancer cells. These treatments are usually given locally, meaning that they are aimed at a particular part of the body where cancer is located. This is different from chemotherapy or other drug therapies, which travel throughout the entire body.

Radiation can be given at several different times during cancer treatment, and for several different reasons. Sometimes radiation is given as a neoadjuvant treatment, meaning before surgery, in order to shrink the tumor and make a successful surgery more likely. Sometimes it's given after surgery, as an adjuvant treatment, to destroy any cancer that is too small to have been removed during surgery. It may be given along with chemotherapy, a treatment approach known as chemoradiotherapy. Radiation therapy is also given as a palliative treatment, meaning that it is used to shrink a tumor so that a person feels better, even though a complete cure of the cancer is not possible. Some examples might be to shrink a tumor causing pain or difficulty breathing or eating.

The most common type of radiation, external beam radiation, is typically given daily on weekdays for a period that could be as short as a single week or as long as two months. The dose of your radiation, as well as the frequency and duration of your radiation treatments, is based on the type of cancer being treated and where it is located in the body, as well as your age and how healthy you are at the time radiation is being given.

This combination of factors is what makes radiation unique as a cancer treatment. It is a local treatment, so it is directed to a specific part of the body and its most intense effects happen in that area. But like systemic cancer treatments such as chemotherapy, which affect the entire body, radiation still has a total-body effect. In other words, even though radiation is usually targeted to one part of your body—where the tumor is located—most patients still feel at least some effect of their radiation treatments throughout their entire body.

Given the differences in radiation dose, treatment schedules, and the location on the body, it is not surprising that people undergoing radiation experience a wide set of side effects, ranging from mild to severe. Many of these are short term, typically related to the area being treated, and are gone a few weeks after treatment ends. A few, however, are longer term, or late side effects, that show up months or even years after radiation was given. Again, the specific side effect often depends on where in the body radiation was delivered.

For example, radiation is very commonly used to treat breast cancer. A short-term side effect in this case could be skin changes similar to a sunburn. Longer-term changes might be a swelling in the arm or chest, known as lymphedema, or damage to the nerves in the arm, causing pain, numbness, or weakness in the shoulder, arm, or hand.

Radiation is used frequently in lung cancer as well. These treatments may damage the lungs and cause a cough, breathing problems, or shortness of breath. Often these improve after treatment, but they don't always go away completely.

Prostate cancer and cancers located on the head and neck are two other types that very often require radiation. When these treatments are given in the prostate region, men may find they have problems going to the bathroom because of damage to the bladder or the bowel. My own father experienced that after his radiation treatments for prostate cancer. Many people given radiation for head and neck cancers get painful sores in their mouth and throat that can make it very hard to eat and drink, leading to weight loss and even malnutrition. My wife, Sara, a head and neck cancer survivor, was only able to eat pancakes—the only food that was not painful to eat—for three weeks near the end of treatment. In addition, lymphedema in head and neck cancer patients can occur in the face, resulting in swollen and tight cheeks. Because the side effects of radiation treatments are so dependent on the dose and cancer location, it is important to talk with your radiation oncologist about how your specific treatments might affect you.

BENEFITS OF EXERCISE DURING RADIATION

The best studies on exercise during radiation have been done in women with breast cancer and men with prostate cancer—two of the most common cancers and two in which radiation is a mainstay of cancer treatment.

There are at least nine "gold standard" randomized controlled trials that have looked at whether exercise helps women with breast cancer undergoing radiation treatment. Depending on the specific study, researchers have compared exercising during radiation treatment with no exercise at all, or compared exercise to a very low-intensity alternative like stretching or relaxation techniques. But overall across all of these studies, which taken together include more than 700 early-stage breast cancer patients, the message was uniformly clear: Regular exercise cut the debilitating fatigue that many patients feel in half.

This same beneficial effect has been shown in prostate cancer. One of the best research groups currently studying exercise in cancer patients, led by my colleague Dr. Kerry Courneya at the University of Alberta in Edmonton, Canada, did a study where they recruited 121 men with prostate cancer and randomly assigned them to a program of resistance exercise, a program of aerobic exercise, or no exercise at all. Importantly, the exercise sessions were manageable: They were done three times a week beginning at only 15 minutes per session. Most people in the study missed at the most only one exercise session every two weeks. And a substantial group—15 percent of men in the study—had enough energy to do additional exercise on their own outside of the study's exercise sessions.

After three months, the results again were clear: Regular exercise, whether it was resistance strength training or aerobic activity, helped reduce fatigue. However, when comparing the two, resistance exercise was even better—the improvements lasted longer and provided additional benefits like more muscular strength and lower body fat. This research study was quite long—these men continued exercising three times a week for six months. But the benefits of exercise are also seen in as little as a few weeks.

Dr. Karen Mustian at the University of Rochester has dedicated her career to studying fatigue in people with cancer. More than ten years ago, she presented work at the world's largest gathering of cancer doctors, the annual meeting of the American Society of Clinical Oncology, showing that just four weeks of daily exercise using a simple at-home program lessens fatigue during radiation treatments and helps preserve muscle strength. She later showed that this same at-home exercise program likely reduced fatigue by helping the immune system adapt to radiation treatment.

This is one of the most promising areas of research on exercise during radiation. My colleague Dr. Zaorsky described it this way: "What we're doing with radiation is using x-rays to cause inflammation in a part of the body. But we know that if you exercise regularly, the inflammation that we see in the blood actually goes down. So the thought is that radiation may cause inflammation in a good way in the short term that acts against cancer, but in the long term, exercise will mitigate the side effects of radiation therapy."

THE PROGRAM:
TRAINING DURING RADIATION THERAPY

We recognize that going through radiation is time-consuming; it's common for appointments to be frequent (often daily). As such, we recommend below a focus on logging, moving, eating, and sleeping, and adding the lift portion of the program as you are able.

LOG

As with chemotherapy, it is crucial to log your symptoms. This is important because it will help you understand the times of day when you have sufficient energy to try an exercise session. The goal is to conserve your energy for the activities that you feel are most important and strike a balance between expending your energy and conserving it—this will allow you to maximize the benefits of exercise without overdoing it.

A good approach is to wake up and prioritize your activities for the day—decide which ones are the most important to you and focus on those. Then think about how best to structure your day. Spread your activities throughout the day and take breaks. If possible, do the most important one first, so that you definitely accomplish it. And whatever the activity, do things slowly, so that you don't use too much energy at once. As with all of the exercise programs in this book, the goal is to maintain regular exercise sessions throughout treatment, not to overdo it and exhaust yourself in the first few sessions.

Log your fatigue/energy level once a day, beginning the day of your first radiation treatment. Your doctor may want you to log other symptoms as well. In your log, record an answer to the following questions:

1. On a scale of 0 (no fatigue) to 10 (most extreme fatigue I've ever felt), how do I feel right now?

2. How did I sleep last night?

3. How much protein did I eat today? (For suggestions on getting enough protein and other nutrition guidance, see chapter 14.)

⟨⊗⟩ MOVE

The recommendation for the move part of the program during radiation therapy is to walk, ideally for 30 minutes a day. While you can certainly do more if you feel well enough and time allows, this recommendation is an acknowledgment of the challenges of completing radiation therapy, logistically and physically.

⟨⊗⟩ LIFT

The lift portion of the program is similar to the one from the chemotherapy chapter. The advice is to lift twice a week to ensure that you avoid the decline in muscle mass that often occurs in cancer patients. The exercises recommended vary according to where you are having radiation therapy.

For example, patients who are undergoing radiation for breast cancer may be too sore to perform upper body strength-training exercises. If so, stop those exercises during the weeks you are receiving radiation treatments. Keep performing the three lower body exercises.

Patients who are undergoing radiation for lung cancer may find themselves too breathless to complete all sets and repetitions of every exercise. Know that there is real value in doing even a single set of each exercise twice weekly.

Regardless of where you are receiving radiation treatments, if fatigue or any other symptoms make it difficult for you to complete the exercises as described, make an effort to do as much as you can—even one session of exercise, only once, is beneficial for your body. Just move. It will help you heal.

Throughout the lift program, you will be doing five exercises. These are the core movements of the lift program. After a day off to assess your body's response, you will add more repetitions to each set. (Recall that a repetition is 1 round of the movement, a set is completing 6 to 10 rounds of the movements described below.) Videos of these exercises can be found at www.movingthroughcancer.com. The recommended exercises are as follows:

....

CHEST PRESS

Lie on your back on a weight-lifting bench, an aerobic step, or on the floor on a towel. Starting with arms straight, bend your elbows to right angles, elbows away from the body, then return arms to straight over your chest. When you add resistance, this will become challenging.

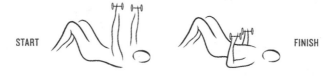

START   FINISH

ONE-ARM ROW

Place one knee and one hand on a chair or the edge of the bed, as shown in the illustrations. Start with your free hand hanging down. Squeeze your shoulder blade toward your spine as you bend your elbow to raise your fist toward your side. Slowly lower to the starting position. Switch and do the other side.

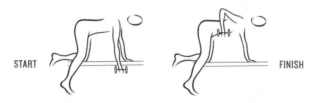

START   FINISH

SQUATS

Stand in front of a full-length mirror, facing to the side. Your feet should be hip distance apart, toes pointed forward. Hold your weights in your hands by your sides (like suitcases), as shown. Sit backward as if you are going to sit down in a chair, keeping your chest lifted, eyes forward. In fact, to start, keep a chair behind you, so that if you touch the chair, you will know you've gone down far enough. Sneak a peek at your knees in the mirror: They shouldn't bend past 90 degrees. Sneak a peek at your knees by looking down: Your knees should not go out past your toes and should stay parallel (not drift toward or away from each other).

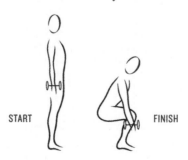

START   FINISH

LUNGES

Hold on to a chair or the wall and step backward with one foot so that you can bend both knees to 90-degree angles, while keeping your chest up. Return to the starting position. Repeat for a full set on one side before switching to the other leg. If you can do lunges without holding on, that's great too. To add resistance for the supported lunge, hold on with one hand and hold a weight in the other hand, at your side.

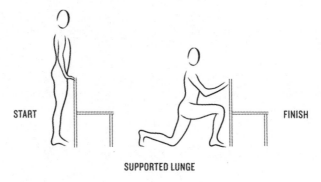

START   FINISH

SUPPORTED LUNGE

DEADLIFTS

Stand with your feet hip-width apart. Bend just at the hips, letting the head follow the back so you are looking at the floor at the end of the movement. Return to standing.

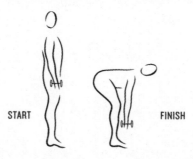

START   FINISH

⊗ EAT

During radiation therapy, you will need to increase your calories and protein so that your body can do the arduous work of killing cancer cells and repairing the healthy tissues that have been affected by the treatments. However, you may develop side effects that make eating more difficult, such as mouth sores or bloating. Bowel habit changes are also common during radiation therapy. If possible, ask for a consultation with a registered dietitian at the facility where you are receiving treatment to get personalized nutrition advice for your particular situation. Overall, the general advice for eating during radiation therapy is to make sure you are getting enough calories and to focus particularly on increasing your protein intake.

☽ SLEEP

The sleep component of the program is the same for both chemotherapy and radiation therapy. The advice is to pay attention to how well you are sleeping, and if you are not sleeping well, to ask for help. Sleep disturbances—whether it be difficulty falling asleep, difficulty staying asleep, or simply waking up tired—are very common during radiation treatments; about half of cancer patients say they have a problem with sleep during radiation.

Yet sleep is crucial for your body to recover from each radiation treatment. If you are not sleeping well, there are non-opioid medications that can be prescribed. You can also apply the strategies outlined in chapter 13 on sleep.

PROGRAM FOR A COMMON RADIATION SCHEDULE
Individual doses and schedules for radiation vary depending on many factors, but it is quite common for cancer patients to receive radiation treatments every weekday for a series of weeks or months. Here's a sample move and lift program for someone receiving four weeks of radiation therapy. Note that each weekend includes both a lift and a move session,

and that lift sessions never occur on consecutive days, which allows the muscles to rebuild after a strength-training session.

Here's a chart of the schedule:

WEEK	MON RADIATION	TUE RADIATION	WED RADIATION	THU RADIATION	FRI RADIATION	SAT WEEKEND	SUN WEEKEND
1	LIFT	MOVE	MOVE	MOVE	MOVE	LIFT	MOVE
2	LIFT	MOVE	MOVE	MOVE	MOVE	LIFT	MOVE
3	MOVE	LIFT	MOVE	MOVE	MOVE	LIFT	MOVE
4	MOVE	LIFT	MOVE	MOVE	MOVE	LIFT	MOVE

PROGRAM FOR COMBINED CHEMOTHERAPY AND RADIATION TREATMENTS

There are a number of types of cancer where combining chemotherapy and radiation and receiving them at the same time is more effective than giving these treatments separately, one after the other. Two common ones include head and neck cancer and certain lung cancers.

People who are given chemotherapy and radiation together very often experience more fatigue and other side effects than they would if they were given these treatments one after the other. In some studies that compare people who get combined chemotherapy and radiation with those who receive only radiation, more than 90 percent of people getting the combined treatment experience at least one moderate side effect. About 60 percent experience a severe one.

As such, if you are receiving these combined treatments, focus on the log, move, eat, and sleep components of the program during this time. If you have energy to do the lift portion of the program for the first few weeks of treatment, by all means do so. But by several weeks into combined chemotherapy and radiation, you are likely to be experiencing a level of fatigue and side effects that simply may not allow you to walk for 30 minutes per day. You will have bad days, but whatever you do, try. Try to walk daily, if you can. As we've said before, no one benefits from sitting on the couch all day. Exercise is the fourth treatment for cancer—do what you can.

Log your symptoms and how they shift over the course of the day to see whether there is a time of day during which it might be possible to walk for up to 30 minutes. If you cannot do 30 minutes, that's OK; do what you can, record it, and try again the next day. Do continue with the eat and sleep portions of the program as well. See the specific chapters on these topics for more details.

WHEN IT IS OVER

One of the biggest shocks for my wife, Sara, and me—and for Dr. Liz O'Riordan as well—was that the symptoms experienced during radiation did not dissipate for weeks after the end of treatment. Sara rang that bell and pounded her fists to the heavens on her last day of combined chemotherapy and radiation. But when she still felt like she could barely get off the couch two weeks later, we realized that it might have been helpful to anticipate that reality. As such, prepare to continue the radiation therapy exercise program plan for about two to three weeks after you are done with radiation therapy. You will recover. It will simply take longer than you may have originally anticipated.

A FINAL WORD ABOUT STIFFNESS

One last word about the effects of radiation and movement. Many patients experience a stiffness in the region where radiation is being received. And while there are no gold-standard exercise oncology studies on this topic, the practical experts in the field, including my friends Regan Fedric and Dr. Karen Wonders from Maple Tree Cancer Alliance, recommend stretching, range of motion, and yoga-type movements to make you feel better as you are going through and beyond radiation therapy. The movements needed are specific to the region being treated with radiation. To see short videos of range of motion exercises that specifically address your situation, see my website, www.movingthroughcancer.com.

HORMONAL THERAPIES

When I talk to people about hormonal therapy, I hear a very common refrain: "I am only fifty-five years old, but I feel more like I'm in my mid-eighties."

They are talking about the joint aches and pains that are a common side effect of hormone therapies, especially when they are first started. Women may also have hot flashes, mood swings, and any number of other changes typically associated with menopause.

And men with prostate cancer, who are also frequently prescribed hormone therapies, are not spared either. They also often feel a number of side effects typically associated with aging: loss of sexual desire, a weakening of the bones, and erectile dysfunction.

Not all people with cancer who are given hormonal therapies feel this way. But many do—in fact, as many as five to eight out of ten patients on these drugs. A lot of these people feel so bad, in fact, that they stop taking their drugs altogether. Some estimates suggest that half of women on aromatase inhibitors stop taking them within two years of starting them. That's a huge number, given that these drugs have been proven to lengthen cancer patients' lives in dozens of studies.

This is the challenge people with cancer and their doctors face: Hormone therapies have a proven benefit against cancers that depend on hormones to grow, but patients have to endure the side effects for a long time to reap the cancer treatment benefits—up to ten years in some cases. You are in it for the long haul. If you're committed to getting the proven survival advantages of hormonal therapies, this is yet one more example of your "new normal" after a cancer diagnosis.

There is a catch-22 at the heart of this challenge: The joint pain and stiffness you may feel while on these drugs can make you think you should not or cannot exercise. But exercise is the very thing that is going to help reduce that pain.

WHAT ARE HORMONAL THERAPIES?

Certain kinds of cancers that we often think of as men's or women's cancers—like breast, ovarian, and prostate cancer—may in some cases be fueled by sex hormones. These hormones, which include estrogen, testosterone, and progesterone, perform many different functions throughout the body, beginning before birth and extending through adulthood. Testosterone, for example, promotes the growth of muscle mass, increases bone density, and is critical to the development of the sex organs in men. The estrogen hormones in women have dozens of functions, from accelerating metabolism and fat stores to blood clotting (to say nothing of the obvious effects women feel when estrogens decline during menopause).

Because of these many functions, sex hormones can also in some cases play a role in the development of certain types of cancers. The cells of these cancers have receptors that serve as docking stations for particular hormones, and when the hormone "docks" on the surface of the cancer cell, it's telling it to grow and multiply. Examples of hormone-receptor cancers include estrogen-receptor (ER) positive and progesterone-receptor (PR) positive breast cancers.

Hormone therapies work by blocking or altering these hormones. By stopping these hormones from attaching to cancer cells, the growth of a tumor can be slowed or even stopped. But because these hormones serve as messengers everywhere from the brain down to the bones in the feet, blocking or altering them has many other side effects. So like chemo-therapy, hormone therapy is considered a systemic treatment—these drugs travel throughout the body seeking out hormones. This is unlike other treatments for cancer that are considered local, such as surgery or radiation, because those treatments primarily affect only the part of the body where the tumor is located.

There have been many studies of hormone therapies done in breast, prostate, ovarian, endometrial, and other cancers. In fact, since 2003 there have been more than a hundred clinical trials published on hor-mone therapies in *breast cancer alone each year.* For more than forty years, hormone therapies have been a mainstay treatment to prevent hormone-dependent cancers from returning and to improve the long-term survival of men and women who have been diagnosed with these cancers. Which hormone therapy your doctor prescribes and when it is used will depend on the type of cancer you have, your age, menopause status if you are a woman, and other aspects of your health and cancer diagnosis.

BENEFITS OF EXERCISE WHILE ON HORMONE THERAPY

Twenty years before Dr. Roanne Segal retired as a medical oncologist to spend more time training for long-distance bike races, she had a question about the hormone therapies she was giving her prostate cancer patients: Could these men, who essentially had no testosterone in their bodies, still build muscle? The question was an important one. When given hormone therapies, both men and women tend to lose muscle and add fat. This phenomenon explained the "pear-shaped" figure she recognized in some of her patients who had been on hormone therapies for a long time. She wanted to know whether strength-training exercises could counteract these changes, even in men who were lacking a major source of muscle building in their bodies.

She put together a research study where half the men who were on hormone therapy for prostate cancer started regularly lifting weights and the other half did not exercise. At the end of the study, she learned two very important things.

"One is that the guys who did no exercise, not only did they lose muscle strength, but they continued to lose it over time. These hormonal therapies are prescribed for years and years, and we learned that it's not 'you lose strength and then plateau.' They lost strength and then they kept losing," she told me when I spoke with her about the study.

The second was that even on these testosterone-blocking therapies, the men who exercised saw a benefit. "The other take-home message was, even though you may have castrate, or extremely low, levels of testosterone, you are still trainable," she said. That is, these men were still able to build muscle mass from a strength-training regimen.

It was unclear why exactly the men who did not exercise kept on losing strength and muscle mass and never really stopped. One theory came to Dr. Segal from observing her patients who didn't exercise: They would lose a little strength and that would make moving just that much harder. They would then do less. The cycle perpetuated itself: A loss of strength meant less movement and less exercise, which in turn led to even greater losses of strength and muscle. "These men correspondingly put on a lot of fat. And so, when that happens, everything you do feels twice as hard. It becomes so difficult to do something; you are fatigued all the time. And so you do less and less over time, which just further exacerbates the situation," she said.

To be clear, many of the negative effects of hormone therapies happen naturally on some level in each of us. Our sex hormone levels peak around the time we have evolved to have children, when our bodies and minds are sharpest so that we can raise our young. But from that point on they start decreasing, albeit relatively gradually. So we all naturally experience a loss of muscle mass and strength, or changes in our brain like forgetting things more often, as we age.

Hormone therapies cause these changes to happen much faster. "These hormonal therapies accelerate the slope of your decline, whether that is the level of your strength or cognitive changes like memory," Dr. Segal said. "Both men and women who are on these therapies have a more precipitous decline as long as they are on them." This is the conundrum of hormone therapy. To reap the cancer treatment benefit, the drugs must be taken for a long time period (up to a decade). However, the side effects can get worse over that long time period.

But this was the key message of Dr. Segal's early studies of hormone therapy: Exercise slowed these declines. The changes were unavoidable on some level—even her prostate cancer patients who exercised lost some strength—but exercise blunted the effect. "Exercise has the ability to mitigate these dramatic changes," she said. "It's not going to fix it completely, but I think it mitigates the precipitous decline for many of the side effects that women and men on hormone therapy complain about."

Studies done since Dr. Segal's original one have borne out her findings, particularly in women diagnosed with breast cancer. For example, several studies have shown that exercise during hormone therapy helps prevent the addition of fat that many women experience on these drugs. Exercise also helps prevent the most common side effect of these drugs, the joint pain and stiffness known as arthralgia, and it is safe to do even if you are already experiencing this arthritis-like pain. Exercise improves brain function generally, and studies suggest that it also specifically helps the cognitive decline that some women experience because of declining hormone levels. Other studies have shown that exercise has a beneficial effect on vitality, social and family well-being, fatigue, sleep disturbances, and body image.

Many of these studies have looked at the quality of people's lives on hormone therapy—in other words, how they feel—which is an important consideration given that you need to be on hormone therapy for two, five, or even ten years to get the most benefit. "Improving quality of life is not an inconsequential outcome," Dr. Segal told me. "And, you know, exercise really has no downside."

THE PROGRAM: TRAINING DURING HORMONE THERAPY

The major difference with the exercise program for hormonal therapy is the length of time you will follow it. All of the previous programs focused on short time periods measured in months: preparing for surgery, recovering from surgery, chemotherapy, and radiation therapy. Each of these likely lasts less than six months. By contrast, hormonal therapy may last up to ten years.

And because hormone treatments last so long, the effects are persistent. To understand the effects of your hormone therapy on your body and mind, it is very important to log how you feel daily. This will help you understand the effects of exercising as well as the effects of not exercising, if you "fall off the wagon" for a time.

In general, the suggested program includes both aerobic activity (move) and resistance exercise (lift). As noted earlier in the chapter, the adverse effects of hormonal therapies fall into many categories: cardiovascular, metabolic, muscular, skeletal, vasomotor (hot flashes), sexual health, cognition, and sleep. It is possible that aerobic activity might be more important for one of these categories (cardiovascular risk) and resistance exercise might be more important for another category (muscular and skeletal health). However, these different types of side effects interact, making a combined program the best one for all outcomes. For example, cardiovascular health risks (for which aerobic exercise might be the first choice) are also affected by metabolic factors and body composition (for which resistance training may be the first choice). As such, it is best that you jump on the combined program bus and ride it out over the years of hormonal therapy. This is a long time period and you may find you want more variety than we can fit into a single book.

LOG

Log your fatigue and energy level and any other symptoms that bother you one time a day. In your log, record an answer to the following questions:

1. On a scale of 0 (no fatigue) to 10 (most extreme fatigue I've ever felt), how do I feel right now?
2. Are there any other symptoms bothering me?
   a. Yes or no
   b. If yes, provide the same 0 to 10 rating for each one.
3. How did I sleep last night?
4. How much protein did I eat today?

 MOVE

The recommendation for the move part of the program during hormonal therapy is to walk, cycle, swim, hike, jog, Zumba, or otherwise get your heart pumping for up to 30 to 60 minutes five to seven times each week. This is a large increase compared with the recommended programs during chemotherapy and radiation, because this recommendation is focused on your cardiovascular and metabolic health, as well as reducing the chances of your cancer coming back.

 LIFT

The lift portion of the program is similar to the one from the prehabilitation chapter. The advice is to lift twice a week to ensure that you avoid the decline in muscle mass that so often occurs during hormonal therapy. After a day off to assess your body's response, you will add more resistance and sets in week two, and continue progressing the resistance over time (see chart starting on page 147). Videos of these exercises as well as other options can be found at www.movingthroughcancer.com. The recommended exercises are on the pages that follow.

CHEST PRESS

Lie on your back on a weight-lifting bench, an aerobic step, or on the floor on a towel. Starting with arms straight, bend your elbows to right angles, elbows away from the body, then return arms to straight over your chest. When you add resistance, this will become challenging.

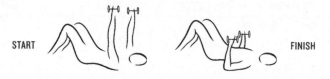

START   FINISH

ONE-ARM ROW

Place one knee and one hand on a chair or the edge of the bed, as shown in the illustrations. Start with your free hand hanging down. Squeeze your shoulder blade toward your spine as you bend your elbow to raise your fist toward your side. Slowly lower to the starting position. Switch and do the other side.

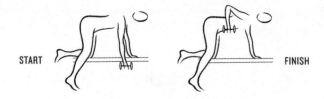

START   FINISH

SQUATS

Stand in front of a full-length mirror, facing to the side. Your feet should be hip distance apart, toes pointed forward. Hold your weights at your sides (like suitcases), as shown. Sit backward as if you are going to sit down in a chair, keeping your chest lifted, eyes forward. In fact, to start, keep a chair behind you, so that if you touch the chair, you will know you've gone down far enough. Sneak a peek at your knees in the mirror: They shouldn't bend past 90 degrees. Sneak a peek at your knees by looking down: Your knees should not go out past your toes and should stay parallel (not drift toward or away from each other).

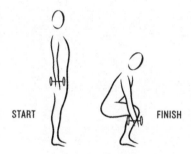

START   FINISH

LUNGES

Hold on to a chair or the wall and step backward with one foot so that you can bend both knees to 90-degree angles, while keeping your chest up. Return to the starting position. Repeat for a full set on one side before switching to the other leg. If you can do lunges without holding on, that's great too. To add resistance for the supported lunge, hold on with one hand and hold a weight in the other hand, at your side.

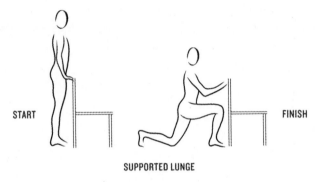

START   FINISH

SUPPORTED LUNGE

DEADLIFTS

Stand with your feet hip-width apart. Bend just at the hips, letting the head follow the back so you are looking at the floor at the end of the movement. Return to standing.

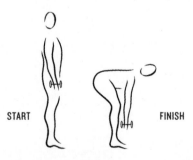

START   FINISH

⊗ EAT

During hormonal therapy, you are at risk of losing muscle and bone mass. Because of this, your diet during hormonal therapy should focus on getting sufficient protein so that any loss is not accelerated by a poor diet. Ask for a consultation with the registered dietitian at the facility where you are receiving treatment to get personalized nutrition advice for your particular situation. Overall, the general advice for eating during hormonal therapy is to make sure you are eating a generally healthy diet and to focus particularly on increasing your protein intake. See chapter 14 for more details on nutrition.

☾ SLEEP

The sleep component of the program is the same for other time points during your treatment. The advice is to pay attention to how well you are sleeping, and if you are not sleeping well, to ask for help. Sleep disturbances—whether it is difficulty falling asleep, difficulty staying asleep, or simply waking up tired—are very common during hormonal therapy.

Yet sleep is crucial for your body and mind to function well. If you are not sleeping well, there are non-opioid medications that can be prescribed. You can also apply the sleep hygiene approaches outlined in chapter 13.

SAMPLE PROGRAM FOR HORMONAL THERAPY

Here's a sample weekly move and lift program for someone receiving hormonal therapy such as androgen deprivation therapy for prostate cancer or aromatase inhibitors for breast cancer. Note that each weekend includes both a lift and a move session, and that lift sessions never occur on consecutive days, which allows the muscles to rebuild after a strength-training session.

Here's a chart of the schedule:

MON	TUE	WED	THU	FRI	SAT	SUN
LIFT	MOVE	MOVE	MOVE	MOVE	LIFT	MOVE

If you prefer to lift and move on the same day, you can double up. This would mean you get two days off from exercise every week.

Below we outline how to progress this program over a two-week period, followed by an explanation of how to increase resistance for the lift program over the course of months and years.

Day 1

Do the five core lift exercises. For each movement, use a level of resistance that matches where you are in your treatment journey, whether you are recovering from reconstructive surgery (light or no resistance) or months out from surgery (heavier resistance).

Do 10 repetitions for each exercise. Use enough resistance to make 1 set of 10 challenging but not overwhelmingly difficult. Use your best judgment—you are allowed to change the weight based on how it goes. (And there will be no quiz at the end.) If you are still recovering from surgery, it is fine to do the session with no resistance. You should also do the eat and sleep components today. Day off from move. Complete the symptom log.

Day 2

Day off from lift exercises. Notice whether and how much your body feels sore from yesterday's session. Be sure to do the move, eat, and sleep components today. Complete the symptom log.

Day 3

Complete the move, eat, and sleep components today. Complete the symptom log.

Day 4

Complete the move, eat, and sleep components today. Complete the symptom log.

Day 5

Complete the move, eat, and sleep components today. Complete the symptom log.

Day 6

Today you are doing the five core lift movements 10 times each. Use the same resistance as the previous lift session. Day off from move. Also complete the eat and sleep components today. Complete the symptom log.

Day 7

Complete the move, eat, and sleep components today. Complete the symptom log.

Day 8

Today you are again doing the core lift movements. In this session, do each movement 10 times for 2 sets (a total of 20 times for each movement). Increase the resistance by approximately 10 percent for each exercise over what you did last week. Sometimes that is not possible depending on the weights or resistance available; if so, increase the weight by the smallest amount possible close to 10 percent. For example, if you were using 10-pound dumbbells for an exercise, you should try to find 12-pound dumbbells for that exercise today. (We know this is a 20 percent increase, but it's hard to find 11-pound dumbbells, so this is as close to 10 percent as you will likely get.) In general, the resistance used for your lower body (squats, lunges, and deadlifts) should be higher than what you do with your upper body (chest press and one-arm row).

When done correctly, you should really be working hard to finish the last few repetitions of each exercise in the last set. If you are not, increase the resistance.

Also complete the eat and sleep components today. No move component today. Complete the symptom log.

Day 9
Day off from lift exercises. Notice whether and how much your body feels sore from yesterday's increase in weight. Complete the move, eat, and sleep components today. Complete the symptom log.

Day 10
Complete the move, eat, and sleep components today. Complete the symptom log.

Day 11
Complete the move, eat, and sleep components today. Complete the symptom log.

Day 12
Complete the move, eat, and sleep components today. Complete the symptom log.

Day 13
Today you are again doing the core lift movements. In this session, do each movement 10 times for 2 sets (a total of 20 times for each movement). Use the same weight you used in the prior session this week. When done correctly, you should really be working hard to finish the last few repetitions of each exercise in the last set. If you are not, increase the resistance.

Also complete the eat and sleep components today. No move component today. Complete the symptom log.

Day 14
Day off from lift exercises. Do the move, eat, and sleep components of the program. Complete the symptom log.

Here's a chart of the program for the first two weeks:

DAY	LOG	MOVE	LIFT			EAT	SLEEP
			SETS	REPS	RESISTANCE		
1	Log symptoms daily to understand whether exercise is making them better	Off	1	10	Post-reconstructive surgery—go light; months since surgery—go heavier	Eat 1.2 g of protein per kg of body weight and hydrate	Prioritize getting 8 hours a night
2		30–60 minutes			Off		
3		30–60 minutes			Off		
4		30–60 minutes			Off		
5		30–60 minutes			Off		
6		Off	1	10	Same as day 2		
7		30–60 minutes			Off		
8		30–60 minutes			Off		
9		Off	2	10	Increase by no more than 10%		
10–12		30–60 minutes			Off		
13		Off	2	10	Same as day 9		
14		30–60 minutes			Off		

This pattern of exercise is repeated for years during hormonal therapy. These are suggestions—you can arrange your exercise time as you see fit, as long as you get 150 to 300 minutes of move and two sessions of lift per week.

To progress the resistance, we suggest that you increase the weight a very small amount for the first session of each week. You can stay with 10 repetitions per set for 2 sets, or you can build to 3 sets if you are motivated to do so. You will be more likely to increase muscle mass with 3 sets over 2. Eventually, approximately six to eight months into the program, you might find that you reach a plateau, where you may not be able to continue increasing the resistance. At that point, it would be worthwhile to identify an exercise professional who can help you design a more advanced program. Try finding one at www .exerciseismedicine.org/movingthroughcancer. Alternatively, check out the short videos, alternative exercises, and other content on my website, www.movingthroughcancer.com.

RECONSTRUCTION

The purpose of this chapter is to support cancer patients who have chosen to undergo reconstruction. The goal is not to guide patients in their decision regarding whether or not to undergo reconstruction but to help patients maintain the best possible physical and emotional well-being as they go through that process. If that's you, read on! If you will not undergo any reconstruction, you can skip to chapter 11.

When I asked my wife, Sara, to look back on her experience with reconstructive surgery, she thought for a moment, and then said: "We had no clue how serious this was going to be."

Ultimately, Sara would have five reconstructive surgeries. As we looked back after each one, we kept realizing how unprepared we had been. We were unprepared for the seriousness of her first reconstructive surgery, an operation known as a "forehead flap," in which the skin of her forehead was folded down and used to reconstruct her nose. From the length of time she'd need to be in the hospital to the level of wound care required once she arrived home, we underestimated it all.

But perhaps our greatest miscalculation was thinking that the surgeries would work differently, better, and easier than they did. With each operation, we held out hope that Sara would wake up with a "normal" nose. Instead, after nearly a half dozen operations, we had to accept that there was nothing more to be done as far as surgery was concerned. There simply wasn't enough tissue to rebuild a functioning nose.

Thankfully, the story ends relatively happily. Two years after her final attempted reconstructive surgery, Sara did get her nose—a beautifully designed prosthetic nose made by a group of artists and engineers who specialize in creating one-of-a-kind artificial body parts.

And while Sara's story is unique in many ways—the number of reconstructive surgeries; the fact that her face was the affected part of her body—in others it's quite similar to what many cancer patients experience when they undergo reconstruction.

The hardest thing for many cancer patients undergoing reconstructive surgery to realize is that it's not a purely cosmetic procedure. The difference between reconstruction and a cosmetic operation is that reconstructive plastic surgeons try to rebuild a part of the body that has been taken apart completely during the surgery to remove the cancer, as compared to a purely cosmetic operation where the surgeon is only enhancing what is already there. In the case of a breast reconstruction, for example, a plastic surgeon is working with breast tissue that has been permanently, irrevocably affected by a previous surgery to remove a cancer.

"The number-one issue that comes up and that we try to stress is that this is reconstruction—we're trying to do it as an aesthetic procedure, but it is not a cosmetic procedure," Dr. Thomas Kinney, a highly regarded reconstructive plastic surgeon in Milwaukee, told me. "There is always going to be something that does not get back to baseline. There are going to be scars. There are going to be areas of the body that we can't make perfect. We do everything in our power to make the body look and feel as natural as possible, but it is still reconstruction."

There are many studies that illustrate just how complicated reconstructive surgery can be. This may be especially true for breast cancer, where the outcome after surgery is deeply entwined with body image, sexuality, and self-esteem. For example, the best and most widely used way to measure how women feel about their breast reconstructions is called the BREAST-Q, a questionnaire that asks women to rate how they feel about their reconstructed breasts from a number of different perspectives, such as how they feel when they look in the mirror or how their bras fit.

Researchers have given thousands of women this questionnaire. On a scale of 0 to 100, the average satisfaction score after surgery, regardless of whether reconstruction was done with an implant or tissue transplant, is typically less than 60 in published studies.

Another study asked women diagnosed with breast cancer how their surgery compared with their expectations. On average, four out of every ten said that the outcome was worse than they expected. About half of these women said it was because of the appearance of their reconstructed breast, most often due to an unnatural appearance and a lack of symmetry between their breasts.

Another common misconception is the length of recovery, Dr. Kinney said. Many people can have a hard time understanding that right after surgery, they are not going to be back to 100 percent strength. Most often it takes at least eight to twelve weeks to feel better after a reconstructive surgery. In some cases, it takes up to a year. Many times patients decide to go back to have additional reconstructive surgery, further stretching their full recovery.

This is due in part to the high rate of complications that can occur after reconstructive surgery. Again looking at breast reconstruction, one in three women has a complication at some point over the following two years. One in five requires more surgery. And for one in twenty, reconstruction fails—meaning they are out of options as far as surgery is concerned.

But this is only one side of the experience, and I highlight it to illustrate that having reconstructive surgery can be complicated. As Dr. Andrea Pusic, chief of plastic surgery and reconstructive surgery at Brigham and Women's Hospital in Boston and the woman who developed the BREAST-Q, told the *New York Times* in 2018, "Choosing reconstruction largely restores satisfaction with your breasts and psychosocial functioning. But it's not uncommon to have bumps in the road."

So remember that study where four in ten women said that their reconstructed breast was less than what they expected? Well, in that study another four of those ten said it met their expectations just fine. And the last two? Their reconstruction was better than they expected.

How you ultimately feel about your reconstruction, whether it is your nose, breast, abdomen, or other part of your body, is a deeply emotional and personal experience. But reconstruction represents something else too, and it's almost always good: Intensive cancer treatment has come to an end. This in itself is an incredible accomplishment—to have gotten through cancer treatment. For so many people diagnosed with cancer, reconstruction is the moment where they get to begin moving on from treatment. They have turned a corner and their whole lives change. Having been through so many procedures and operations, chemotherapy and radiation therapy, they now realize that they are getting better. Cancer treatment is going to eventually be behind them. They are going to be able to get on with their lives.

"From an emotional, psychological, and physical standpoint, these people are putting their cancer behind them at this point because in their minds, that's done," Dr. Kinney told me. "Most people don't want to continually think about their cancer. So undergoing reconstruction puts them in a whole different mindset. They tend to put their diagnosis aside for now and concentrate on the reconstruction."

Even my wife Sara, whose experience was difficult, found that she turned a corner during the experience. In her case, it was an emotional corner. As I mentioned in chapter 2, Sara had for the most part been a shy, introverted person; she once told me she wanted to "go through life unnoticed." Walking around in public for two years as her nose gradually disintegrated during round after round of reconstructive surgery, she was noticed in ways she could never have imagined. In shops or around town, every single person she passed looked at her—and she knew why. "I looked back at myself and I thought, 'Really, I wanted to go through life unnoticed?'" She was forced to face the idea that maybe she could be living a better way. "I really began to uncover my authentic self," she said.

For all of these reasons—physical, emotional, and psychological— exercise is critical after reconstructive surgery, whether the goal is to have the best outcome or take back control of your life after cancer treatment. Exercise can reframe the whole story by helping you focus on what your body can do, rather than how it looks.

A BREAK FROM THINKING ABOUT CANCER

So let's focus on what you can do during and after your reconstructive surgery, not on how you look. Because reconstructive surgery by definition involves repairing damaged tissues in the body, a lot of reconstructive surgery patients find they have issues with their movement or range of motion after surgery. To use breast reconstruction as an example, regardless of the type of reconstructive surgery you may have, whether it is an implant or autologous tissue transplant, your strength and movement will very likely be compromised immediately after the operation. In the case of implants, the effects will be in the upper body, around the shoulder and arm. In the case of a tissue transplant, you may have issues in your upper body as well as the donor site where your tissue was taken from, often the abdomen.

The good news is that exercise helps restore this physical function, and for many people who have lingering effects after reconstruction, it speeds the recovery process. Most reconstructive surgeries change the way that muscles are recruited to do physical work like lifting, carrying, or pushing. After a reconstructive surgery, your body will try to correct for these changes; in doing so, you may begin to recruit muscles that were not meant to perform those actions and actually upset the balance between muscle groups over the long term. Doing the exercises included in this chapter will help your body use the right muscles to do the daily work of lifting and carrying, preventing any lasting negative changes. If your abdominal wall has been affected, perhaps because tissue was taken from your stomach to be transplanted into your reconstructed breast or elsewhere, these exercises are critical for strengthening your core, the foundation for nearly all of our daily movements.

Range of motion exercises may be even more important. These movements prevent your muscles and other tissues from contracting and keep them flexible during the recovery from surgery.

Physically, exercise is clearly important. But for many patients, this actually pales in comparison to the incredible sense of empowerment they feel by exercising as they put intensive cancer treatment behind them. Similar to how exercise improves your chances of finishing treatments and beating cancer, we now have dozens of high-quality studies showing that exercise improves the way that people with cancer feel. When you look at the results of these studies collectively, which include thousands of patients, the results are irrefutable: People who exercise consistently say that they feel better physically and emotionally and that they have stronger social connections with their friends and families.

It's hard to prove exactly why this is, though my colleague Dr. Kerry Courneya has a hypothesis that makes a lot of sense. Exercise has plenty of easily measurable effects, such as reducing blood pressure and increasing muscle strength. These are the ways that exercise likely helps with the physical side effects of cancer treatment—in other words, exercise reduces the occurrence of symptoms.

But exercise also does many other things that are harder to measure. For one, it distracts you. Nearly every patient I've spoken with tells me that exercise "gives them a break from thinking about cancer." When you're walking vigorously or lifting weights, it is really difficult to focus on the anger or anxiety you may be feeling about your diagnosis. And if you are interacting with family or friends when you exercise, such as a group exercise class or walking with a partner or an exercise buddy each day, then you are distracted that much more as you pay attention to someone else. In this way, exercise interferes with symptoms—you are not focusing on them because you are thinking about something else.

The last part has to do with spiritual well-being—and this is the part that connects with reconstruction. It has to do with finding meaning and purpose in your life. Exercise is the best way to take back control of your body. It is also intrinsically linked to feelings of hope and pride. You are driven to exercise because you see potential in your future—putting your cancer treatments behind you, getting on with your life, and feeling healthy and energetic again.

Dr. Kinney sees this with his patients and I've seen it over and over again in my research studies as well. I've also seen it personally with my wife, Sara. Early on, she was very angry with her diagnosis and her treatment. And she had no outlet for it. Then she found boxing. I do not like boxing—it is not my thing—but I went with her to help get her going. She's quite small, maybe 120 pounds soaking wet, but my God, I have never seen her go at it like she does in the gym. Physically, emotionally, spiritually—that's where she lets go of her anxiety, anger, and frustration: in the boxing ring.

THE PROGRAM:
TRAINING DURING RECONSTRUCTION

Throughout reconstruction, you will cycle between the program from chapter 5 (prehabilitation) and the program from chapter 6 (recovery from surgery) until you are done with the repeated surgeries sometimes needed for reconstruction. Once complete, you can continue to chapter 11 (post-treatment). This assumes you will not be undergoing chemotherapy or radiation therapies in between your reconstructive surgeries.

There is one other element of the program that is needed as you traverse the reconstruction zone: evaluation from a qualified rehabilitation health professional (physical or occupational therapist, physiatrist, or rehabilitation nurse) and, if they deem it appropriate, cancer rehabilitation. Earlier in the chapter we mentioned range of motion and abdominal strength changes as examples of what patients might experience during the process of reconstruction. The specific exercises to do—as well as avoid—to improve those issues are highly personal and are best evaluated and prescribed by a rehabilitation health care professional. Ask for a referral to physical therapy from your reconstructive surgeon if you are not automatically referred. And follow the home program recommended by your physical therapist in addition to following the program described in this section for the best possible results. If no such specialist exists or you have no insurance coverage for cancer rehabilitation evaluation and treatment, please use the guidance available on my website, www .movingthroughcancer.com.

Many readers will have been diagnosed with breast cancer, and we recognize that the reconstruction process for breast cancer is distinct from other types of reconstructive surgery. The program that follows is intended for all patients undergoing reconstruction, but we specifically checked in with oncology physical therapist Dr. Leslie Waltke, from the Facebook group The Recovery Room, and we are confident that what follows is appropriate for breast reconstruction of both types: free flaps and implants.

SURGICAL RECOVERY PHASE

Reconstructive surgery, whether it is of the breast, nose, colon, esophagus, or a limb, is still surgery. If you are going under general anesthesia, it is surgery. As such, the surgical recovery program from chapter 6 is appropriate for the weeks following reconstructive surgery until your surgeon clears you to lift weights again.

PREPARATION FOR YOUR NEXT
RECONSTRUCTIVE SURGERY

Once your surgeon has cleared you to lift weights, you can start to prepare for the next reconstructive surgery, if there is to be one. To do so, return to the prehabilitation program from chapter 5. Sara had five reconstructive surgeries, so she did this loop from surgical recovery to prehabilitation five times. Each patient is unique. It is possible that there may be no additional surgery for some who undergo immediate reconstruction with a free-flap surgery. If this is you, skip this next section—it is for patients who have an additional reconstructive surgery to undergo.

The prehabilitation program focuses on five areas: log, move, lift, eat, and sleep. See chapter 5 for details. If you have been prescribed physical therapy sessions, consider those sessions and the associated home program a sixth area.

After you have surgery, move back to the beginning of the program for recovery in chapter six. Once you have completed recovering from surgery, move to the next chapter—congratulations, it's time to put major cancer treatment behind you!

II

POST-TREATMENT

F inishing cancer treatment is an incredible accomplishment. It is likely that few people in your circle of family and friends will truly understand what you've been through—the anxiety and frustration that can come with a cancer diagnosis, the deep fatigue and other side effects that accompany treatment. Successfully completing cancer treatment is rightly a time for celebration.

And yet, along with that celebration often comes a sense of "What now?" and a recognition that there are likely effects of cancer treatment that will linger for quite some time. Fatigue is the main one—many people with cancer keep experiencing some level of the fatigue they felt during treatment even after it's over. A loss of muscle strength is also common, especially for breast cancer and prostate cancer survivors who were given hormone therapy. This loss of strength can really interfere with your daily life.

The point is this: To the outside world, it might look like cancer is behind you. And for the most part it is. But there is a good chance that you are probably going to have some lingering effects in at least one area of your life.

The incredibly good news is that there are now hundreds of research studies that have shown that exercise improves both the physical and the mental recovery after cancer treatment is over, and that it can prevent and improve the lingering side effects that can persist. So yes, it is possible to get back to where you were physically and mentally before your diagnosis.

Bill Jollie's story illustrates well the anxiety and depression you can feel after cancer treatment. It also shows the beneficial—even transformative—power of exercise.

Four years into remission, the deep fear that basically all cancer survivors have came true for him—one day in the shower he noticed an enlarged lymph node. He'd had a particular kind of lymphoma that often recurred, so he was pretty sure this was going to happen at some point, he just didn't know when.

Five months into treatment he was in a bad place. The targeted therapy that he was on left him feeling deeply fatigued—a constant lack of energy and purpose that had accumulated into melancholy and was on its way to becoming full-blown depression.

Known to friends as "Jollie," Bill is one of most gregarious and positive people I've met. That he was feeling this low is a testament to what cancer can do to even the most high-spirited people. "I didn't want to talk to my wife or to my daughters; I didn't want to go to work. I would just watch TV and go to bed early. I was in a really deep hole," Bill told me of that time. He thought he might have to stop treating his cancer just so that he could prevent the clinical depression he felt sure was coming on.

One Thursday night after a week of particularly bad days, Bill decided to go for a jog, not to "get healthy" but simply to clear his mind—"to figure out how I could get out of this," he told me.

Once he got going, something happened: His entire mood—in fact, his entire outlook—changed. "A mile into my run, that whole weight lifted—the despair, the depression. It put me on a new path. And what I found out in the months after that was that if I went a few days without exercising, those feelings would creep in again," Bill said.

"I found that exercise can alter the way I'm feeling and alter the way I think," he added. "When you are a cancer patient, everything is being done to you. You lose all control over your body. Exercise and diet are ways to gain control back, to be able to say, 'I am actively fighting my cancer.'"

At this point, Bill's experience has been borne out in almost too many medical studies to count. The science in this area is unequivocal: Exercise is safe and effective for cancer survivors. It improves cardiovascular fitness and strength and has positive effects on fatigue, emotional well-being, and the overall quality of survivors' lives.

Let's look specifically at fatigue, since it is the most common side effect of cancer treatment, it has the biggest negative impact on people's lives, and it often persists long after treatment stops. In fact, as many as one in three cancer patients have low energy, concentration, or motivation—the hallmarks of fatigue—well into their lives as cancer survivors.

What actually causes this fatigue is complex and not entirely understood. But scientists believe that the chronic inflammation caused by cancer and its treatments is a very likely explanation for at least a substantial part of it. And we know that exercise reduces inflammation. In fact, levels of at least a half dozen cytokines—the proteins our immune system releases to increase inflammation when fighting cancer or healing from treatments—are lowered when we exercise.

Regardless of whether scientists know exactly why it happens, we know exercise works. When researchers collect all of the studies that have looked at exercise and fatigue in cancer survivors, the benefits are clear. And this includes more than one hundred studies and 100,000 cancer survivors, as well as many different modes of exercise, from walking and strength training to yoga, Qigong, and Tai Chi. This stands in stark contrast to drug treatments, which have little to no effect.

But this perhaps misses the most important point of all: Exercise reduces the likelihood of cancer coming back. Observational studies that compare sedentary and active cancer survivors have consistently shown that moving more decreases cancer recurrence. Just as one example, when researchers looked at more than 12,000 survivors of breast cancer, they found that exercising reduced the chance of their cancer coming back by 24 percent. Other studies have shown this to be true for colorectal, ovarian, lung, brain, and prostate cancers as well.

My colleague Dr. Christine Friedenreich follows this question—whether exercise after treatment prevents cancer from returning—more closely than any other exercise researcher in the world. She keeps a database where she collects information from all of the studies on this topic, and she updates her database each time a new study is published. She most recently updated her database in 2018, at which time it included data from 136 studies. The results are unequivocal: Cancer survivors of all types studied who exercise are 37 percent less likely to die of cancer. (And, as a bonus, are 39 percent less likely to die of any other cause, like heart disease or a stroke.)

When she updated the data, Dr. Friedenreich also looked closely at the "dose" of exercise in each of these studies. What she found, not surprisingly, is that more exercise is better than less. But very importantly, she also found that the greatest benefit came in the transition from a completely sedentary lifestyle to exercising just a little bit. Going from no exercise at all to just 2 hours a week provides a much greater relative improvement in health than going from 10 hours a week to 12.

It is not simply that exercising is good. Not exercising at all is actually bad. This may be intuitive, but studies have looked specifically at what a sedentary lifestyle does to cancer survivors. When researchers from the American Cancer Society surveyed more than 2,000 colorectal cancer survivors, they found that longer leisure time (nonworking time) spent sitting was associated with a higher risk of death. Other studies have shown that being sedentary as a cancer survivor affects your mood as well, contributing to more feelings of fatigue, depression, confusion, and even anger.

Finally, even if you've been completely inactive up until this point, don't beat yourself up—instead, get moving! It is still incredibly beneficial to get started right now. We know this from the Women's Health Initiative, one of the largest women's health projects ever launched in the United States. In this study, women with breast cancer who exercised after their diagnosis—even when they were completely inactive before it—showed improvements in their ability to remain cancer free as a survivor.

The most important point is to begin, regardless of your fitness level or whether or not you have exercised before. As Dr. Jeff Meyerhardt, who codirects the Colon and Rectal Cancer Center at the Dana-Farber Cancer Institute in Boston, put it to me: "Doing some is better than none. Try to get up to 150 minutes per week, but if you only have time or the tolerance to do 75, that's undoubtedly better than being inactive. Start slow with 5 or 10 minutes per day for the first week and then slowly build up. See where you can get to. If it doesn't get back to exactly where your prior levels were before cancer, or what your expectations are, that's OK. Just give it time."

THE PROGRAM: TRAINING DURING POST-TREATMENT

The exercise program for the period after your treatment is designed to be followed for years, or even decades. This is distinct from previous chapters that focused on short time periods of weeks or months: preparing for surgery, recovering from surgery, chemotherapy, and radiation therapy. Each of these prior time frames likely lasted less than six months. By contrast, the post-treatment time frame is, hopefully, for the rest of your life. The goal is to get into a regular habit, and then to move on and live, thrive, and, hopefully, watch your cancer experience disappear in the rearview mirror.

To understand your progress and track improvements in the symptoms and side effects that may linger after treatment, it is advisable to keep filling in your log. Once a day is sufficient. This is important because it will help you understand the effects of exercising and the effects of not exercising, if you "fall off the wagon" for a time.

In general, the suggested program includes both aerobic activity (move) and resistance exercise (lift). As noted earlier in the chapter, the adverse effects of treatment do not simply disappear the day you ring the bell or stop taking hormonal therapy. Further, the types of adverse effects that linger interact with one another, making a combined aerobic and resistance-training program the best one for all outcomes. For example, cardiovascular health risks (for which aerobic exercise might be the first choice) are also affected by metabolic factors like your cholesterol level and body composition (for which resistance training might arguably be the first choice). As such, it is best to combine aerobic and resistance exercises during your years after treatment.

LOG

One time per day, log your fatigue/energy level and any other symptoms that bother you. In your log, answer the following questions:

1. On a scale of 0 (no fatigue) to 10 (most extreme fatigue I've ever felt), how do I feel right now?

2. Are there any other symptoms bothering me?
   a. Yes or no
   b. If yes, provide the same 0 to 10 rating for each one.

3. How much and how well do I sleep at night? Sleep quality matters as much as quantity. This is subjective. Perhaps rate your sleep for the prior night on a scale of 0 (didn't sleep/slept horribly) to 10 (best night of sleep you've ever had). For more on sleep, see chapter 13.

4. How much protein did I eat today? You are aiming for 1.2 grams per kilogram of body weight. (For suggestions on getting enough protein and other nutrition guidance, see chapter 14.)

MOVE

The recommendation for the move part of the program is to walk, cycle, swim, hike, jog, Zumba, or otherwise get your heart pumping for up to 30 to 60 minutes five to seven times each week. This is a large increase compared to the recommended programs during active treatment because you are now focused on your cardiovascular and metabolic health, as well as reducing the risk of your cancer recurring.

LIFT

The lift portion of the program should be familiar by now, as we've tried to stay consistent throughout the book. The advice is to lift twice a week to ensure that you rebuild your muscle and bone mass after treatment. After a day off to assess your body's response, you will add more resistance and repetitions in week two, and continue progressing the resistance over time. Videos of these exercises and possible alternative exercises can be found at www.movingthroughcancer.com. The recommended exercises are as follows:

....

CHEST PRESS

Lie on your back on a weight-lifting bench, an aerobic step, or on the floor on a towel. Starting with arms straight, bend your elbows to right angles, elbows away from the body, then return arms to straight over your chest. When you add resistance, this will become challenging.

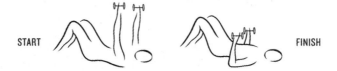

START   FINISH

ONE-ARM ROW

Place one knee and one hand on a chair or the edge of the bed, as shown in the illustrations. Start with your free hand hanging down. Squeeze your shoulder blade toward your spine as you bend your elbow to raise your fist toward your side. Slowly lower to the starting position. Switch and do the other side.

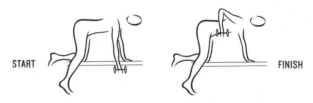

START   FINISH

SQUATS

Stand in front of a full-length mirror, facing to the side. Your feet should be hip distance apart, toes pointed forward. Hold your weights at your sides (like suitcases), as shown. Sit backward like you are going to sit down in a chair, keeping your chest lifted, eyes forward. In fact, to start, keep a chair behind you, so that if you touch the chair, you will know you've gone down far enough. Sneak a peek at your knees in the mirror: They shouldn't bend past 90 degrees. Sneak a peek at your knees by looking down: Your knees should not go out past your toes and should stay parallel (not drift toward or away from each other).

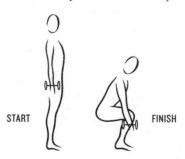

START   FINISH

LUNGES

Hold on to a chair or the wall and step backward with one foot so that you can bend both knees to 90-degree angles, while keeping your chest up. Return to the starting position. Repeat for a full set on one side before switching to the other leg. If you can do lunges without holding on, that's great too. To add resistance for the supported lunge, hold on with one hand and hold a weight in the other hand, at your side.

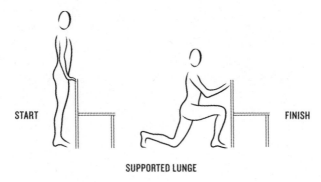

START   FINISH

SUPPORTED LUNGE

DEADLIFTS

Stand with your feet hip-width apart. Bend just at the hips, letting the head follow the back so you are looking at the floor at the end of the movement. Return to standing.

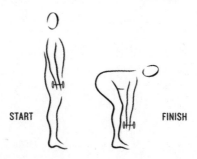

START   FINISH

EAT

Post-treatment, you finally have the opportunity to regain any muscle mass and bone that might have been lost during treatment. As such, one focus of your diet in the time frame after treatment should be to ensure that you have sufficient protein intake to build muscle and bone. If possible, ask for a consultation with the registered dietitian at the facility where you are receiving treatment to get personalized nutrition advice for your particular situation. See chapter 14 for overall nutrition guidance.

(☾) SLEEP

The sleep component of the program is the same for other time points during your treatment. The advice is to pay attention to how well you are sleeping, and if you are not sleeping well, to ask for help.

Sleep is crucial for your body and mind to function well. If you are not sleeping well, there are non-opioid medications that can be prescribed. You can also apply the sleep hygiene approaches outlined in chapter 13.

PROGRAM FOR POST-TREATMENT

Here's a sample weekly move and lift program for someone who recently completed treatment. Note that each weekend includes both a lift and a move session, and that lift sessions never occur on consecutive days, which allows the muscles to rebuild after a strength-training session.

Here's a chart of the schedule:

MON	TUE	WED	THU	FRI	SAT	SUN
LIFT	MOVE	MOVE	MOVE	MOVE	LIFT	MOVE

If you prefer to lift and move on the same day, you can double up. This would mean you get two days off from exercise every week.

Below we outline how to progress this program over a two-week period, followed by an explanation of how to increase resistance for the lift program over the course of months and years.

Day 1

Do the five core lift exercises. For each movement, use a level of resistance that matches where you are in your treatment journey, whether you are recovering from reconstructive surgery (light or no resistance) or months out from surgery (heavier resistance).

Do 10 repetitions for each exercise. Use enough resistance to make 1 set of 10 challenging but not overwhelmingly difficult. Use your best judgment—you are allowed to change the weight based on how it goes. (And there will be no quiz at the end.) If you are still recovering from surgery, it is fine to do the session with no resistance. You should also do the eat and sleep components today. Day off from move. Complete the log.

Day 2

Day off from lift exercises. Notice whether and how much your body feels sore from yesterday's session. Be sure to do the move, eat, and sleep components today. Complete the log.

Day 3

Complete the move, eat, and sleep components today. Complete the log.

Day 4

Complete the move, eat, and sleep components today. Complete the log.

Day 5

Complete the move, eat, and sleep components today. Complete the log.

Day 6

Today you are doing the five core lift movements 10 times each. Use the same resistance as the previous lift session. Also complete the eat and sleep components today. Complete the log.

Day 7

Complete the move, eat, and sleep components today. Complete the log.

Day 8

Today you are again doing the core lift movements. In this session, do each movement 10 times for 2 sets (a total of 20 times for each movement). Increase the resistance by no more than about 10 percent for each exercise over what you did last week. Sometimes that is not possible depending on the weights or resistance available; if so, increase the weight by the smallest amount possible close to 10 percent. For example, if you were using 10-pound dumbbells for an exercise, you should try to find 12-pound dumbbells for that exercise today. (We are aware that's a 20 percent difference, but it is rare to find 11-pound dumbbells, so that's likely the smallest increase from 10 pounds.) In general, the resistance used for your lower body (squats, lunges, and deadlifts) should be higher than what you do with your upper body (chest press and one-arm row).

When done correctly, you should really be working hard to finish the last few repetitions of each exercise in the last set. If you are not, increase the resistance.

Also complete the eat and sleep components today. No move component today. Complete the log.

Day 9

Day off from lift exercises. Notice whether and how much your body feels sore from yesterday's increase in weight. Complete the move, eat, and sleep components today. Complete the log.

Day 10

Complete the move, eat, and sleep components today. Complete the log.

Day 11

Complete the move, eat, and sleep components today. Complete the log.

Day 12

Complete the move, eat, and sleep components today. Complete the log.

Day 13

Today you are again doing the core lift movements. In this session, do each movement 10 times for 2 sets (a total of 20 times for each movement). Use the same weight you used in the prior session this week. When done correctly, you should really be working hard to finish the last few repetitions of each exercise in the last set. If you are not, increase the resistance.

Also complete the eat and sleep components today. No move component today. Complete the log.

Day 14

Day off from lift exercises. Do the move, eat, and sleep components of the program. Complete the log.

Here's a chart of the program for the first two weeks:

DAY	LOG	MOVE	SETS	REPS	LIFT RESISTANCE	EAT	SLEEP
1	Log symptoms daily to understand whether exercise is making them better	30–60 minutes			Off	Eat 1.2 g of protein per kg of body weight and hydrate	Prior-itize getting 8 hours a night
2		Off	1	10	Post-reconstructive surgery—go light; months since surgery—go heavier		
3		30–60 minutes			Off		
4		30–60 minutes			Off		
5		30–60 minutes			Off		
6		Off	1	10	Same as day 2		
7		30–60 minutes			Off		
8		30–60 minutes			Off		
9		Off	2	10	Increase by no more than 10%		
10		30–60 minutes			Off		
11		30–60 minutes			Off		
12		30–60 minutes			Off		
13		Off	2	10	Same as day 9		
14		30–60 minutes			Off		

This pattern is repeated for years during the post-treatment time frame. These are suggestions—you can arrange your exercise time as you see fit, as long as you get 150 to 300 minutes of move and two sessions of lift per week.

To progress the resistance, we suggest that you increase the weight a very small amount at the first session of each week. You can stay with 10 repetitions per set for 2 sets, or you can build to 3 sets if you are motivated to do so. You will be more likely to increase muscle mass with 3 sets over 2. Eventually (likely six to eight months into the program), you might find you reach a plateau, where you may not be able to continue increasing the resistance. At that point, it would be worthwhile to identify an exercise professional who can help you design a more advanced program. Try finding one at www.exerciseismedicine .org/movingthroughcancer. Alternatively, go to my website, www .movingthroughcancer.com, for additional options.

SURVIVORSHIP

Whether you view yourself as a cancer survivor is entirely up to you. For many people with cancer, or who had cancer in the past, being a cancer survivor is a badge of honor—they have made it through one of the most difficult challenges of their lives. Others may view themselves as survivors in the sense of being part of a larger group of advocates working for better research and treatment on behalf of others with cancer. Still others would never think of themselves this way. After all, we do not call those who suffer heart attacks "cardiovascular disease survivors," do we?

Regardless of how you define yourself after treatment, cancer today should not be viewed as a death sentence—far from it. Two out of every three cancer patients live at least five years, and one out of every five lives more than twenty years. For some cancers, like stage 1 breast cancer, survival past five years is approaching 100 percent. In fact, many people with some of the most common cancers—like colorectal, prostate, and breast cancer—have a higher risk of dying from some other medical condition than any form of cancer. Most frequently, it's heart disease.

That is why it is important to continue moving long after you finish treatment. Most people diagnosed with cancer today can expect to live well into old age. Regular movement will not only add to these years, but it will also make them more enjoyable. And very importantly, as we will discuss later in this chapter, regular exercise reduces the likelihood of your cancer returning.

YOUR OWN RESILIENCE CAN BE VERY POWERFUL

At age twenty-four, Dr. Keith Bellizzi found himself facing something completely unexpected: a stage 3 testicular cancer diagnosis. Three months later, doctors told him he also had an unrelated kidney cancer. While most people his age were either whiling away their youth or starting their careers, Dr. Bellizzi was suddenly faced with his own mortality. "I had a lot of time to reflect on where I was in life, where I wanted to go, and what my purpose would be in life. That was the catalyst that changed my entire life trajectory," he told me.

He made a promise to himself and his family: If he survived, he would quit his job, go back to school, earn a PhD, and dedicate his life to better understanding the lives of cancer survivors. And this is precisely what he has done, including training at and later working for the Office of Cancer Survivorship at the National Cancer Institute. Personally and professionally, Dr. Bellizzi has witnessed how surviving cancer changes someone. And he has both studied and lived the choices that can make life after cancer richer and more fulfilling.

What he has seen is that resilience is more the norm than the exception. "Most people do not realize what they are capable of until they are put into a life-threatening situation. When I think about my own experience, I had no other choice but to fight."

This can be incredibly empowering: Step back and realize, first and foremost, that you have gotten through something incredibly difficult—something that perhaps at times you didn't think you would. Perhaps you got through it with grace and courage. Perhaps you feel you just made it through by the skin of your teeth. Either way, recognizing your own resilience can be very powerful.

A lot of people find the process of cancer treatment life changing. When they finish, they take a step back and look differently at what lies ahead. I also spoke with Dr. Bellizzi's mentor at the National Cancer Institute, Dr. Julia Rowland, former director of the Office of Cancer Survivorship, who has spent her career helping cancer patients live better lives after treatment. She added that many people find the experience of getting through treatment very "permission giving." They tend to concentrate on the most meaningful aspects of their life and commit to not taking them for granted for anymore. At the same time, they look at things that have caused grief or sorrow and give themselves permission to let go of them.

For Dr. Bellizzi, this experience was his chance to find his purpose in the world. "I would say that cancer was one of the best things that happened to me. And I truly believe that, because I would not be in the position that I'm in without that experience. I have been able to make a difference and help a lot of people who have gone through similar experiences."

However, not everyone feels this way. And having a positive attitude or finding a "silver lining" should never be expected. The late Dr. Jimmie Holland, arguably the most influential psychiatrist in the history of oncology, spent her career arguing against the "tyranny of positive thinking"—the notion that cancer patients have to be positive about their outlook to ensure the best outcome. This pressure to stay upbeat all the time—often placed on cancer patients by well-meaning loved ones—can actually make dealing with the difficulties of cancer even harder. The ways that people cope with adversity are completely unique to them, based on their DNA, their temperament, and their life experiences. There is no place for judgment about how you feel about getting cancer or surviving it.

WHAT'S GOING TO HAPPEN NOW?

Despite the accomplishment of making it through, finishing treatment can be cruelly ironic, in a way: Having been through months, or even years, of grueling treatments, one of the greatest challenges can actually be concluding your relationship with your cancer care team.

"I still remember my five-year appointment with my oncologist quite vividly. He completed his exam, reached out to shake my hand, and said, 'Congratulations, you've successfully completed the treatment protocol and I no longer need to see you.' You would think that this would have been a moment of great relief and joy," Dr. Bellizzi told me. "In fact, it was the exact opposite. As I walked out of his office, the nurses lined the hallway and clapped and cheered for me. But once I was out in the waiting room, I felt like I had been punched in the gut."

Until that point, every six months Dr. Bellizzi's oncologist would reassure him that his cancer was in remission. Who would be giving him that peace of mind—telling him that everything is OK? "I just felt like I lost a huge part of my support system."

In her decades of work with cancer survivors, Dr. Rowland has also seen this as a crisis moment for some who have come through the other side of cancer treatment. When you are in treatment or under surveillance, there is often the sense of just trying to get through one day at a time. But once you are completely done with that, there is no schedule and often no plan either. Struggling to make sense of "life after cancer," many people wonder, "What's going to happen now?"

One difficult lesson some learn during this period is that cancer, in the meanest way possible, is a gift that keeps on giving—the difficulties do not end just because treatment and visits with your oncologist are done. These difficulties are called "persistent" or "late effects" of cancer treatment. It's quite common for side effects like fatigue to linger; but it is less well known that issues related to cancer treatment can pop up five, ten, and even twenty years after the end of treatment.

There are really four different types of these late effects: physical, psychological, social, and existential spiritual effects.

On the physical side, fatigue, "chemo brain" and other cognitive issues, lymphedema, and post-surgical pain are common persistent side effects of treatment. But perhaps the most serious long-term effect of cancer treatment is cardiovascular disease. Cancer treatments ranging from chemotherapy to radiation can cause a wide range of heart issues, which tend to develop slowly over time. Anthracycline chemotherapies in particular are known for causing heart failure. One key to managing this risk is surveillance, whether that is by your oncologist, primary care doctor, or cardiologist. And the other key is—you guessed it—exercise. We have decades of evidence clearly demonstrating that exercise is one of the best ways to reduce the risk of heart disease.

Long-term psychological effects of cancer treatment can include bouts of acute or chronic depression and anxiety. These can take many forms, from difficulty concentrating or sleeping to unexplained trembling and feelings of detachment from oneself or the world around you. In fact, one form of post-treatment anxiety is experienced by essentially all cancer survivors: fear of their cancer returning. When this anxiety peaks just before follow-up appointments or surveillance scans, it's called "scanxiety." When I studied this particular form of post-treatment anxiety with colleagues at the University of Pennsylvania, we found that the overwhelming majority of lung cancer patients we surveyed felt particularly anxious around their scan appointments and it didn't change even when they had recently had a good scan result or were further out from finishing treatment. For some cancer survivors, it never goes away. "I'm twenty-five years out from my first diagnosis and I still have anxiety," Dr. Bellizzi told me. "Anytime I go to the doctor, I still have anxiety. Whenever I experience a strange new symptom, the first place my mind goes to is, you know, is my cancer back?" There can be many other triggers, even idiosyncratic ones like the smell of rubbing alcohol or needle sticks. Perhaps the anniversary of your diagnosis or driving by the hospital causes anxiety.

Social effects have to do with relationships with your family and friends. It is very likely that you drew closer to a handful of people throughout your treatment—they were the ones who were really there for you. There were probably even one or two who came completely out of the blue, people you never expected would be delivering meals or driving you to appointments. But it is also possible that a couple of your relationships are now more distant. This can happen when someone you expected to really be there for you during a difficult time in fact wasn't.

Finally, it is very common for cancer patients to wonder why they got cancer, especially if there are no clear predisposing factors like a genetic mutation or family history. Sometimes people who have been diagnosed with cancer question God as a result. This is a common spiritual long-term effect of cancer.

The question then is, how do you manage these issues if and when they come up? Between them, Drs. Bellizzi and Rowland have spent decades working with cancer survivors and they have recognized what helps people thrive in this new chapter of their lives.

Acknowledge that these things may be coming. Recognizing that you might experience some of these late effects of treatment is half the battle. Preparation makes a big difference. Recovery is going to take a while—it can be helpful to think of it as "one day in, one day out." In other words, a rough estimate is that recovery will take as long as treatment. However long it takes, give yourself permission to heal—not only your body, but your mind and spirit as well. Treatment happened to everything—your emotional, social, and spiritual well-being, too—and all that needs mending and rebalancing. Resist the expectation that everything is going to just slide right back to normal. If it does not, that can be very stressful and cause anxiety and depression for some people, especially if they are not aware it is coming. If you feel it would be helpful, you can also tell your friends and family to expect some of these changes even after treatment is long over so that their expectations are realistic as well.

Cultivate resilience. Part of Dr. Bellizzi's research has looked at what makes individuals resilient in the face of adversity. "What we know is that resilient people focus on what is within their control. There are a lot of things that are outside of our control, but resilient people engage with the meaningful, controllable aspects of their lives rather than ruminate about the uncertainty of their disease."

One approach is simply reframing a situation. If you are feeling particularly anxious in the run-up to a surveillance scan, for example, it can be helpful to reflect on your track record of getting through difficult times. So far, it's 100 percent—that's pretty darn good!

You also have control over how you respond. There are many techniques to regulate the emotions that accompany stress, beginning with simple breathing exercises. Evidence-based mindfulness and meditation apps available on your phone are a great way to begin.

Finally, look for healthy support systems and resilient role models. Cancer support groups, both online and in person, can be really good for finding resilient role models who understand and empathize with your personal situation. Similarly, if you are feeling particularly unsettled about some aspect of your cancer history, don't turn to people who are fatalistic or tend to catastrophize situations.

Move more. Exercise is particularly helpful as a cancer survivor. As we mentioned earlier, there are decades of data demonstrating that exercise is incredibly beneficial for heart health. It will also help reduce the long-term cardiotoxic effects of chemotherapy and radiation. As we have talked about throughout the book, exercise is also great for reducing anxiety—after all, you can't worry about an upcoming scan when you are pushing through the final reps of a strength-training set or race walking up a hill! And exercise remains the very best intervention medicine has for fatigue from cancer treatments.

But the one benefit of exercise that we have not expanded on much—but likely the most important one for cancer survivors—is that it reduces the likelihood of your cancer returning. While it has been shown in studies of prostate and colorectal cancer as well, the best evidence we have comes from women with breast cancer. In these women, regular physical activity has been consistently linked with a lower risk of breast cancer recurrence. One of the key messages from these studies is that you do not have to go overboard. The minimum recommended amounts of exercise can have a dramatic effect. In one recent analysis that collected data from sixty-seven previous studies, just 30 minutes of exercise five times a week led to a 40 percent reduction in breast cancer recurrence. In another, walking for at least 1 hour a week at a very manageable pace (about 25 minutes per mile) led to clear reduction in the chances of breast cancer coming back, especially once the study participants got four or five years out from their initial diagnosis. The exercise in these studies was not intense; it was moderate exercise that can be incorporated into everyday life, like brisk walking, dancing, or cycling. The take-home message is that simple daily walking can have an outsized impact by reducing the chances of your cancer returning.

We also have good—and growing—evidence that exercise will improve the long-term side effects of treatment that we mentioned above, like fatigue and anxiety. But there are some things exercise may or may not help with—there just is not scientific evidence for it at the moment. And we don't want to sell you on anything that is not based in science.

For example, it is not uncommon for cancer patients who received chemotherapy during their treatment to feel tingling or burning sensations, or numbness and weakness, in their hands or feet. This is caused by damage to the nerves outside the brain and spinal cord and is called peripheral neuropathy. In this area, the evidence that exercise is beneficial is emerging, but not as solid as some of the other areas we've discussed. It will help you in all of the others that we mentioned, but if you are suffering from debilitating nerve pain, we just can't say with certainty that exercise will help.

The same is true for sexual health, which is very commonly affected in men and women who have had cancer in the sex organs. There is emerging evidence that exercise might have a positive effect on sexual activity in men with prostate cancer, and we know that exercise is beneficial for sexual health in the general population, but it has not been as firmly established as the other benefits of exercise we outlined earlier.

MAKING A PLAN, FINDING YOUR MOTIVATION

What separates this phase of your journey as a cancer survivor from the others you have experienced so far is that most cancer survivors can expect to live a long time. Unlike surgery or chemotherapy, your life as a survivor of cancer is almost certainly going to be measured in years, not weeks or months. So there is likely going to be a point, or several, in which you "fall off the wagon" when it comes to regular exercise.

First, this is OK—expected, even. You are going to have bad or "off" days. You are absolutely going to have days when you do not want to exercise. On some of these days, hopefully you push through and follow the "10-minute rule": walk, jog, or do some other moderate-intensity exercise for 10 minutes and see how you feel. If you feel better, continue on; if you feel noticeably worse, then stop for that day. You might take a day off or even a couple of days, knowing that tomorrow is a new day and that you will wake up with a different mindset.

I also spoke with Dr. Sherry Pagoto, a psychologist from the University of Connecticut who specializes in developing good lifestyle habits to reduce cancer and heart disease, about how to get back on track. The following are her suggestions.

Have a plan for "falling off the wagon." Do not hold yourself to the unreasonable expectation of perfect exercise habits for the rest of your life. Make a plan for what you are going to do when you miss a few days. It might be that you start off easy again, at half your regular distance; lay out your workout clothes for the next day before you go to bed; or sign up for a class at the gym. Having this plan puts you back in control. Dr. Pagoto has noticed that the people who are really successful when it comes to changing their lifestyle over the long term tend to be totally OK when things go wrong with their workouts or diet. They slide through moments of adversity without getting too hung up on where they went wrong.

Avoid black-and-white thinking. Be careful not to fall into the mental trap of thinking that a lapse once or twice is a reason to give up completely. Let us be clear: It is not. This shift in thinking will give you some permission and forgiveness if you miss a day or two, but then pick up and get back to your plan as quickly as possible.

Find a community. You are likely to be more accountable if you are exercising with someone else. Whenever possible, get moving with an exercise partner. You will be far less likely to give up if you know that your spouse or friend is counting on you, or if you are a regular in the workout class at your gym. If you need help finding an exercise buddy, reach out to 2unstoppable.org. Alternatively, find an accountability partner—someone you check in with regularly but you don't actually exercise with.

Revisit your motivations. Hopefully when you read chapter 4 you spent some time thinking about your motivations for exercising. (And if not, that's fine too. Now is also a great time to get them down on paper.) Go back and reread them. Think about how you felt in that moment—remember your purpose and that exercise is going to help you achieve it.

You are now on the other side of an enormous journey through cancer treatment—probably one of the most challenging periods of your life. This is something to celebrate!

One of the big lessons that many survivors learn is that there is a rich and wonderful life to be had after cancer treatment. In some ways, it may even be richer than your life prior to cancer. And one of the best ways to get your mojo back after this life-altering journey is exercise. Remember: Just keep moving. Keep on moving. Physical activity is pretty much everything you do every day when you are not sitting down. It is walking around the house, going up and down the stairs, doing laundry. It is mowing the lawn and raking the leaves. It is walking the dog. It all counts and it is all helping you in many different ways.

THE PROGRAM:
TRAINING FOR THE REST OF YOUR LIFE

The program here is the exact same program as in chapter 11, which discussed exercising immediately after treatment. Like that chapter, as well as certain long-term treatments like hormonal therapies in breast cancer, this is a program that is meant to be followed for years, or even decades. See chapter 11 for the program. In general, the suggested program includes both aerobic activity (move) and resistance exercise (lift). As noted earlier, the adverse effects of treatment do not simply disappear the day you ring the bell or stop taking hormonal therapy. Further, the types of adverse effects that linger interact with one another, making a combined aerobic and resistance-training program the best one for all outcomes. For example, cardiovascular health risks (for which aerobic exercise might be the first choice) are also affected by metabolic factors like your cholesterol level and body composition (for which resistance training might arguably be the first choice). As such, it is best to combine aerobic and resistance exercises during your years after treatment.

Further, post-treatment, you finally have the opportunity to regain any muscle mass and bone that might have been lost during treatment. As such, one focus of your diet in the time frame after treatment should be to ensure that you have sufficient protein intake to build muscle and bone. If possible, ask for a consultation with the registered dietitian at the facility where you received treatment to get personalized nutrition advice for your particular situation. See chapter 14 for overall nutrition guidance.

We also recognize that you may eventually want more variety. Go to www.movingthroughcancer.com to find more exercise ideas and learn about programs near you.

PART THREE

SUPPORTS AND SUCCESSES

SLEEP

Has this ever happened: You wake up in the middle of the night, and even though you are desperate to fall back asleep it's just not coming? Eventually, you crack and look at the clock. Now the thinking starts: *It's 3 A.M.—I've been awake for an hour. If I fall asleep right now, I'll still get five hours.*

Of course you don't fall asleep "right now" because your mind has fully woken up. It may even have kicked into overdrive, worried about how a night of terrible sleep is going to affect your workday tomorrow or the list of tasks you needed to accomplish.

If you are reading this book because of a recent cancer diagnosis, then there is about a one in two chance that you've experienced some variation of the above night, not once or twice but with some regularity. Cancer tends to affect older people, in whom sleep problems are much more common. And if you're any younger, you're dealing with the classic stressors of middle age: professional pressures, raising children, perhaps taking care of your own aging parents.

In order to get into what causes sleep issues and how they can be fixed, it is important to understand exactly what we're talking about when we say "sleep problem."

During and after cancer treatment, when we mention sleep disturbances, we're talking about insomnia. The field of sleep science includes anatomical causes of disrupted sleep like sleep apnea, sleep-related movement disorders such as restless legs syndrome, and biological causes like thyroid hormone imbalances. The field of sleep science is much broader than insomnia, but insomnia is the most prevalent sleep issue among people who have been diagnosed with cancer. This is what we are focusing on in this chapter.

If one of the above anatomical or biological issues is causing your sleep disturbance, then following the advice throughout this chapter will help rule out other causes and make it easier to get the help you need to resolve the underlying issue.

So what constitutes an insomnia problem? We have all had sleep issues from time to time. A disrupted schedule might throw you off for a few nights or nerves could have you tossing and turning before a big day. But when sleep specialists talk about sleep problems, they have specific criteria. For this chapter, I spoke with Dr. Sheila Garland, a psychologist who focuses on sleep issues in cancer patients and with whom I worked at the University of Pennsylvania. Dr. Garland told me that insomnia means difficulty falling asleep at the beginning of the night for more than 30 minutes and/or lying awake during the middle of the night for more than 30 minutes, with this happening at least three nights a week for three months.

If some of this sounds familiar, it is because it is incredibly common after a cancer diagnosis. The rate of people showing symptoms of insomnia in the general population is about 10 percent. At the time of a cancer diagnosis, it is 60 percent, a percentage that includes people who had symptoms of insomnia before they found out they had cancer as well as those who are not sleeping well because of the news of their cancer diagnosis. Of these 60 percent, 28 percent meet the criteria outlined above for insomnia disorder. This goes down to about 20 percent a year and a half after diagnosis, but that is still twice as much as the general population.

A cancer diagnosis is a trigger for insomnia, but treatment itself is horrible for sleep as well. For example, we have strong research showing that with each successive round of chemotherapy, your circadian rhythms become progressively disrupted. Your circadian rhythm serves as the "clock" of your body, more or less, and plays a part in everything from your appetite and mood to your memory, concentration, and attention. When researchers attach Fitbit-like devices to cancer patients undergoing chemotherapy, what they find is that with each cycle of chemotherapy, the person tends to be become less active during the day and more active during the night, which is probably the result of disrupted sleep. During intensive treatments, people are more likely to nap during the day, or to be sedentary and lying around on the couch, for example, and this impacts the length and the depth of sleep at night.

When it comes to sleep, one of the biggest problems with chemotherapy is that it is often given with corticosteroids. Two of the most common are prednisone and dexamethasone. These drugs have beneficial effects during cancer treatment, including lowering inflammation, reducing feelings of nausea and vomiting after a round of chemo, and improving your appetite. What is often not mentioned to patients is that these medicines are very activating. In fact, they are so stimulating that some people feel euphoric after a dose. More routinely, people on steroids simply feel very awake and therefore have poor sleep while they are on them. Although your doctors may not mention this side effect when giving you steroids, it is important to keep in the back of your mind so that if you do experience problems sleeping, you can place them in context, recognizing that the steroids you are taking are probably the cause of your restless nights.

During treatment, it can be hard to separate the feeling of fatigue that very commonly comes with cancer treatment from the tiredness that comes from not sleeping well. But there is a simple test to separate the two. Ask yourself, "If I laid down and closed my eyes, would I fall asleep?" More often than not, with fatigue the answer is no. The mind is still active, even though the body feels physically depleted.

You can also separate the two by looking at trends over longer periods in your log. Put simply, fatigue likely will not be helped by more sleep. In other words, cancer-related fatigue is not really dependent on, or proportional to, what you do during the day. You can have good sleep, or try to be very restful throughout the day, and you will still probably feel very tired if you're suffering with cancer-related fatigue. But if you're sleepy, that will be corrected by sleep. You will feel better and be more active after nights of good sleep, and this will be reflected in your log book.

Being chronically underslept, yet still having to function in daily life, is obviously its own kind of private hell. And no insomniac needs a reminder of how awful this feels. But even beyond just feeling crummy all the time, chronic insomnia has multiple downstream effects that are important to understand as you undergo cancer treatment. There is very strong evidence, for example, that insomnia can actually predict a depressive episode. People with insomnia are more likely to develop cancer-related fatigue. Insomnia is linked to the forgetfulness and difficulty concentrating that many cancer survivors refer to as "chemo brain." There is even some evidence to suggest that insomnia increases the risk of infections during chemotherapy and may even make chemotherapy less effective.

The bottom line is that even though you may have placed incredible emphasis on diet and exercise before, during, and after cancer treatment, you are not going to be able to do either of these things well if you are not sleeping.

Sleep Hygiene Tips

- Have a fixed wake-up time.

- Get outside in the sunlight.

- Be physically active.

- Limit naps to 30 minutes and nap no later than the early afternoon.

- Keep your bedtime routine consistent.

- Dim your lights in the evening.

- Avoid alcohol.

- Unplug from electronics at least 30 minutes and ideally 90 minutes before sleep.

- Lower your thermostat at night to around 65 degrees Fahrenheit.

- Block out light with heavy curtains or an eye mask.

- Drown out noise with earplugs, a fan, or a white noise machine.

- Meditation, mindfulness, paced breathing, aromatherapy, and other relaxation techniques can help as you wind down.

- If you haven't fallen asleep after 20 minutes, don't toss and turn. Get up and stretch, read, or do something else calming before trying to fall asleep again.

The good news is that sleep can absolutely be improved, even in the weeks after a cancer diagnosis and throughout the months and years of treatment that follow. The go-to, gold-standard treatment for insomnia is a non-drug approach known as cognitive-behavioral therapy. It has the most solid evidence for anybody who has insomnia, whether they are a cancer survivor or someone in the general population. In studies, it works for about 60 percent of people with chronic insomnia: 30 percent of people who follow through with cognitive-behavioral therapy get rid of their insomnia completely; in the other 30 percent, their symptoms improve—meaning they get more and better sleep—but they still have some nights of difficult or poor sleep. And for the remaining 40 percent of people with insomnia who try cognitive-behavioral therapy in research studies, they either do not complete the treatment or it doesn't work for them. Again, these results are as good as medications over the short term and even better than drug treatments over the long term.

Very briefly, cognitive-behavioral therapy focuses on challenging unhelpful thoughts or beliefs to see whether they are actually true. It is a coping mechanism that helps place our fears and anxieties in context.

I will give a very common example, one my colleague Dr. Garland hears often when treating people with chronic insomnia: "If I don't sleep tonight, tomorrow is going to be horrible." The anxiety will be specific for you, whether that's stress around a big meeting with your boss the following day or the fear that you will have bags under your eyes and everybody will be able to tell immediately that you did not get any sleep last night. But the template is the same: You are not sleeping and that is going to have catastrophic consequences.

The first step in cognitive-behavioral therapy is looking closely and identifying this core belief or thought. Put another way, what do you actually fear will be the consequence of not sleeping?

Then you do a little calculation and test this out. To keep with the work example, many people feel that their professional life is going to fall apart because of chronic insomnia. Hypothetically, let's say that you have insomnia on average three or four nights a week—a significant amount to be sure, but still a moderate case of insomnia syndrome. This means that you're underslept 182 days a year—or half the time. You then reflect: Has my work life fallen completely apart? Have I been fired?

The answer is no, your professional life has not completely fallen apart. That is the thing about these unhelpful thoughts: They are rarely true. In fact, you have been functioning—perhaps not at your peak, but you have been coping with this problem of insomnia. It is far from ideal, but the worst-case scenario that you've been envisioning has not happened, even over the course of months and months of insomnia.

This is just an example. At its root, cognitive-behavioral therapy is about revising these very personal and specific thoughts and fears with more realistic statements. In essence, with cognitive-behavioral therapy, you are recognizing that your worst fears—the ones that literally keep you up at night—are not true and will not come true.

This approach is very well studied, and not only for sleeping disorders. It has been shown to be as effective as drug therapy for less severe forms of depression, anxiety, post-traumatic stress disorder, substance abuse, and eating disorders.

Cognitive-behavioral therapy works because it disrupts a feedback loop at the root of insomnia: Worrying about sleep is the very thing that causes you to have problems sleeping. Conversely, the less you worry about sleeping, the more likely that your sleep is going to recover.

As we noted earlier in the list of sleep hygiene tips, there are a number of other things that you should do to support healthy sleep during cancer treatment. The first is to have a consistent wake-up time. The moment you wake up is the most important anchor of your circadian rhythm because it determines your bedtime. And your wake-up time should not change regardless of how much or how little you slept during the night or what day of the week it is. So even if you got really crappy sleep the night before, get up at your usual time. This in turn means that your sleepiness, or sleep pressure, is going to be very, very strong at the end of the day and you are more likely to have better sleep the following night.

Here is a related problem that sometimes affects people undergoing cancer treatment: They've been going to bed at midnight and waking up at 7 A.M. to get to work for years. That is, they are 7-hour-a-night sleepers. But when they are off work, either undergoing treatments or in between them, they no longer have that pressure to get up at 7 A.M. So then maybe they start sleeping in until 9 A.M.—yet they still want to go to bed at 12 A.M. because that's when they've always gone to bed. But you do not just become a 9-hour-a-night sleeper when you have been a 7-hour sleeper for most of your adult life.

When you sleep in, you move that "wake-up anchor" later and you actually push your bedtime that much further out. So now, rather than falling asleep at 12 A.M., this person now lies awake until 2 A.M., when they begin their habitual 7-hour sleep cycle.

There is not a great deal of difference between getting 7 hours of sleep starting at midnight versus 2 A.M. But what often happens is that this person lies in bed for those 2 hours wondering, *Why am I not sleeping?* And when that happens, night after night after night, they start to develop an association between their bed and being awake. A classic example of this is feeling sleepy or even falling asleep on the couch, but then going to bed and finding yourself feeling wide awake. This can be corrected by a regular, enforced wake time.

Another strategy to correct insomnia is to match your sleep ability to your sleep opportunity. The log you keep throughout treatment is helpful here. Let's say you are recording only 5 hours of sleep a night, even though you are spending 10 hours in bed (because you are desperate for sleep). Rather than lying in bed for all this time awake, only spend 5 hours in bed. Pick a reasonable wake-up time and work backward: If 6 A.M. makes sense to start your day, then go to bed at 1 A.M.

This is absolutely frightening for most people. The idea of being in bed *less* when you want to sleep *more* is completely counterintuitive. But right away you are maximizing your body's pressure for sleep—a nice way of saying that you are so tired when you finally crawl into bed that you fall asleep.

The approach helps people fall asleep quickly, but just as importantly they also fall asleep deeply and they stay in deep sleep longer. So even though they are still sleeping the same amount—5 hours in this example—their sleep is more consolidated and they feel better because of that.

Some sleep scientists call this "leaving out the wake time" and it is a way of retraining a person's body and mind how to sleep again. Without the time spent lying awake wondering why they are not sleeping, a strong association between being in bed and sleeping has been restored. With each successive week, a bit more sleep time can gradually be tacked on.

There are many sleep hygiene tips that are widely available online; we've provided you with a list of those that have a scientific underpinning. Most of these tips focus on following a nightly routine and optimizing your bedroom for sleep. They are all important, but the one that Dr. Garland emphasizes to her insomnia patients—the one that bears repeating—is to implement a 90-minute, device-free buffer zone before bed. Getting away from backlit devices like televisions, laptops, and phones and into a relaxing, non-stimulating environment in dim light is very important.

This is a book about exercise, so you might wonder: How does regular exercise effect sleep? There is sound evidence that regular exercise supports good sleep. In research studies, daily walking, regular strength training, and yoga have all been shown to have a positive effect on sleep in people with cancer. There are also many studies demonstrating that regular exercise helps sleep in the general population. Exercise reduces anxiety, which may contribute to better sleep. Exercise may also help shift and establish circadian rhythms.

That said, there are a couple of important things to keep in mind about exercise and sleep. The first is that timing matters. It is thought that one of the ways exercise impacts sleep is through body temperature, which is closely tied to sleep onset and depth. If you exercise in the evening, that can have a direct impact on the body's ability to rev down because anything that gets your core body temperature up can confuse your circadian rhythm. It is best to exercise in the morning, but also fine to do so in the afternoon if that is the time that works. Exercise in the evening and at night should be avoided if possible.

Another caveat is that while exercise supports good sleep and has been shown to improve sleep quality and shorten the time it takes to fall asleep, it is not a cure-all for sleep problems. This is because many of the thoughts and behaviors that lead to sleep problems are not addressed by exercise alone. Exercise is hugely beneficial for overall health as well as for dealing with cancer specifically, but if you have underlying causes for poor sleep, those should be addressed in conjunction with regular exercise.

One of the important things about getting these habits, and your sleep, on track is that it allows you to separate out some of the negative side effects of cancer treatment. If your sleep habits are strong and you are getting the recommended 7 to 9 hours a night, then you can definitively identify feelings of fatigue as cancer-related, as opposed to sleep-related. This is important because the treatments for each are different. If you are getting good total sleep time, but are still excessively sleepy during the daytime, it could be a sign of an underlying undiagnosed sleep disorder like obstructive sleep apnea or a sleep-related movement disorder. To address these disorders, find a sleep specialist. You might start with your general practitioner or oncologist to identify a sleep specialist.

Getting your sleep right is also uniquely beneficial during cancer treatment: Every aspect of recovery during cancer treatment—from wound healing after surgery to mental health and cognitive functioning long after treatment is over—will be enhanced by proper sleep. And good sleep is crucial to being able to adhere to the exercise regimen recommended in other chapters of this book.

If you have taken these steps and still find that you are not sleeping well, there are drug treatments that your doctors can prescribe, even beyond the well-known sleep drugs like Ambien. It is important to remember that unlike good sleep hygiene, regular exercise, and the cognitive-behavioral approach of reframing unhelpful thoughts around sleep, these drugs all have side effects, most notably drowsiness. But if you're struggling with sleep, it is very important to get it resolved, even if it may mean medication or a combination of medicine and other approaches.

Many people take over-the-counter or "natural" sleep aids. Mention any of these that you are taking to your oncology nurses and doctors. These are considered nutritional supplements by the Food and Drug Administration. That means they are not required to undergo the same rigorous testing as prescription medications. And very importantly for people with cancer, their long-term side effects and possible interactions with other drugs are often not known.

Finally, if you are wondering whether to prioritize sleep or exercise during your treatment, look at your log. If you are getting 7 to 8 hours a night of good-quality sleep, prioritize your exercise. If you find you are unable to sleep well or for that long and it is interfering with your functioning during the day, prioritize getting your sleep sorted out first, then come back to the exercise. Sleep is that important.

NUTRITION

When you are being treated for cancer, eating becomes a part of your medical plan. Of course, you still want to enjoy your food (to the extent that it is possible for you) and the sense of community that eating with others can bring, but for the period of time during active treatment, in particular, you want to think about your diet as a way to support your treatment. In exactly the same way that surgery, chemotherapy, and radiation—and exercise—will help you beat your cancer, what you eat is also a part of your treatment regimen. Put very simply, cancer patients who maintain good nutrition during treatment are more likely to be able to handle the side effects of treatment.

And like exercise, this is also a part of the treatment plan that you are responsible for. Your doctors will be treating your cancer in the most effective way they can. Your caregivers will be responsible for supporting you. But your food choices—like exercise—are an important aspect of cancer treatment that is more within your control than, say, the choice of chemotherapy regimen.

Eating during cancer treatment can be difficult, even painful at times. But it can also be an amazing opportunity, from witnessing the help and support of others to becoming a more adventurous shopper in the grocery store and more confident cook in the kitchen, regardless of prior experience.

BUYER BEWARE

Let's begin by saying that there is a lot of misinformation on the internet about nutrition and cancer. I spoke at length for this chapter with my colleague Dr. Cynthia Thomson, who is a professor in the College of Public Health and holds joint appointments in the College of Agriculture and Life Sciences and the College of Medicine at the University of Arizona, and she put it as follows: "It's almost scary to send them out into that world, because there are a lot of supplement companies trying to make money on cancer patients."

Thus, it's really important to recognize what a healthy diet can and cannot do for you during cancer treatment. There is scientific evidence, for example, that maintaining good nutrition can help reduce side effects of treatment, prevent delays in getting treated, and help maintain your overall well-being throughout treatment. These benefits are important because they help you get through cancer treatment successfully.

However, diets and nutritional supplements are not cancer therapies in and of themselves, and changes to your diet should not be looked at as a way to enhance your treatments or target the cancer itself. The internet is rife with wellness quacks peddling specific diets—or worse, specific supplements or blends—with supposed cancer-fighting benefits. Be wary of any information that claims a particular diet or dietary supplement can improve your prognosis after you have been diagnosed with cancer—as we will outline, in some cases certain diets or supplements may even worsen your response to treatment.

But that does not mean you shouldn't change your diet after a cancer diagnosis. In fact, anywhere from 30 to 85 percent of people diagnosed with cancer lack proper nutrition. Before we get into how to improve your diet before and during treatment, a few definitions are called for. There are many different ways to describe a lack of proper nutrition, or malnutrition, but for cancer patients the primary aspects are as follows: insufficient energy intake, weight loss, loss of muscle or loss of the fat just beneath the skin, and macronutrient deficiencies. When we talk about macronutrients, we're essentially referring to types of food, like carbohydrates (breads and cereals), proteins (meat and beans), and fats (salad dressing and butter).

One of the most common macronutrient deficiencies among older people—including those who get diagnosed with cancer—is a lack of protein. Several of the largest nutritional studies done to date—including the National Health and Nutrition Examination Survey and the Women's Health Initiative—have found that only about 50 percent of older Americans get enough protein in their diet. This is the primary reason why we focus on protein intake elsewhere in this book.

Counterintuitively, obesity can actually mask this type of malnutrition—that is, one can be overweight but still lacking in essential macronutrients. We also know that body mass index—the most common rule of thumb for determining whether someone is underweight, average weight, or overweight—is not really good for determining nutrition status either.

So regardless of weight, someone can be metabolically unhealthy, meaning that their blood pressure, cholesterol, blood sugar, and triglycerides put them at risk of heart disease, diabetes, and other metabolic diseases. As Dr. Thomson told me, "The assumption is that people who are obese are eating unhealthy, and people who are lean are eating really healthy. And that is so untrue."

Cancer can be a specific case in point. People diagnosed with cancer have often lost a lot of weight recently. That might be considered a good thing, but if you've lost weight under the condition of cancer, without following a healthy diet and exercising, you have likely lost a lot of muscle along with fat. This can make cancer treatments harder to endure—this loss of muscle has been linked with experiencing more side effects that are also more severe. These more frequent and more intense side effects can in turn lead to reducing treatment doses or pausing or stopping treatment altogether, which not surprisingly affects how well the treatments work.

IMPROVING YOUR NUTRITIONAL
HEALTH DURING CANCER

We know that if you start off treatment healthy and then you do things to further enhance your nutritional health, you are more likely to have a better outcome. The question then is, how do you improve your nutritional health? The reality for many people with cancer is that they are not going to get specialized nutrition advice from their care team unless they actively seek it out. It is, unfortunately, simply a numbers game: Research done by the National Cancer Institute has shown that registered dietitian nutritionists are not routinely employed in the outpatient cancer centers where more than 90 percent of all cancer patients are treated. Put another way, there is one registered dietician nutritionist for every 2,308 cancer patients in the United States. This is an average, meaning that there are even fewer nutrition specialists in rural or underserved areas.

Most of the nutrition advice you receive in the cancer center will be driven by your oncologist and whether they feel nutrition is relevant to the care of their patients. To that end, ask to be screened for any nutrition risks. If the screening tool—usually one of several simple questionnaires—shows that you are at risk, ask if you can receive a more comprehensive nutritional assessment. Ideally, you would also ask your oncologist to measure for vitamin D, anemia, and other nutritional markers that are relatively cheap to test for and reimbursable through insurance.

You can also take steps on your own to assess your current nutritional intake. The simplest and most straightforward way to track your diet is using an app on your phone. One of the most popular is MyFitnessPal, though there are many others. Most of these use either crowdsourced nutrient data or nutrient data from third parties, meaning some apps have incomplete data. Practically speaking, this might mean that if you look at the nutrient data for a Fig Newton, for example, it might show that it has 3 grams of fiber without mentioning that it also has 9 grams of added sugar. So when choosing an online or a phone-based diet tracker, look for one that uses reliable sources, such as the USDA nutrient database. See my website for ideas on reliable trackers (www .movingthroughcancer.com).

If you are interested in using a more comprehensive tool, the National Cancer Institute offers the ASA24, or Automated Self-Administered 24-hour Dietary Assessment Tool. This tool is frequently used by researchers and physicians, but it can also be used by patients who are looking for a more sophisticated—but also more complicated—tool to track their dietary intake. It can be found online at Epi.grants .cancer.gov/asa24.

One of the issues with most dietary trackers is that they often take a snapshot of your diet, rather than providing a broader picture. Even the ASA24—as the name itself attests—only tracks your diet for a 24-hour period. But because your diet changes on a day-to-day basis, a much better approach is to look at your diet over a two- to three-week period. If there is one element to take away from this chapter, it would be this: A healthy diet is about a *pattern* of intake, and in particular a pattern of choices that is rich in fruits and vegetables, is high in fiber and protein, and avoids processed foods. If you eat in this way over time, you are not going to have micronutrient deficiencies in specific vitamins or minerals because the pattern will provide comprehensive nutrient intake.

As an example, the recommended daily amount, or RDA, of vitamin C is 75 to 90 milligrams per day. Following a diet that prioritizes fruits and vegetables might mean you get 60 milligrams one day, but that you get 110 milligrams the next. When you follow this dietary pattern, you do not need to worry about hitting specific RDA values on a daily basis—over time you maintain healthy nutrition.

The plant-based Mediterranean diet is an ideal pattern of healthy eating. It has been incredibly well studied by researchers and its benefits are firmly established. Follow it if you can and you like the food. But there has also been a recognition that not everyone wants to eat food from the Mediterranean region. Thankfully, there are a number of culturally appropriate, heritage dietary plans that take the basic framework of the USDA food pyramid and apply it to African, Latin American, and Asian foods. One source is Oldways (oldwayspt.org), a nonprofit that offers simple dietary plans and recipes based on these principles but adapted to cultures from around the world. At the end of the day, the basic approach remains the same: Whatever cultural culinary tradition you choose to eat from, try and move toward a plant-based diet that prioritizes protein, which is very important when you are fighting cancer.

If you look around for a diet that appeals to you, especially online, you will undoubtedly encounter advice—often with the goal of selling you something—that advocates a particular diet or blend of supplements specifically tailored for its cancer-fighting properties. The idea that a particular diet can enhance your response to cancer treatment cannot entirely be dismissed out of hand. For example, the ketogenic diet—a low-carbohydrate, high-fat diet that reduces the amount of sugar in your bloodstream—is currently being studied in brain cancer patients with glioblastoma.

But this next, very important point cannot be overemphasized: This research is very early, much of it has been done in mice, and it is not applicable to the larger group of cancer patients yet. On the contrary, what we do know with certainty is that the more restrictive your diet is, the more likely you are to have macronutrient deficiencies. So while you can certainly achieve proper nutrition with more restrictive approaches like vegetarian, vegan, or ketogenic diets, you will need to be that much more vigilant about making sure you are getting the recommended amount of macro- and micronutrients like protein and vitamins and minerals from other whole-food sources.

Beyond moving toward a plant-based diet generally, the primary specific dietary concern for people with cancer is getting enough protein. As stated above, this is why we focus on protein in the rest of this chapter. The loss of muscle that many people experience during cancer treatment has real effects on their outcome and overall health. And the only way to maintain and build muscle using the resistance exercise programs throughout this book is by eating sufficient protein. Particularly during cancer treatment, you should be thinking about protein intake at every meal, with the goal of getting 1.2 grams per kilogram of body weight over the course of each day. For the average person weighing 75 kilograms

(165 pounds), this would equate to two eggs at breakfast, a cup of cottage cheese at lunch, 2 ounces of cheese for a snack, and 6 ounces of salmon at dinner. If this sounds like a lot of food, or not reasonable based on your current appetite, please know there are high-quality protein supplements on the market. Some are powders that you can mix into your own choice of milk, water, juice, or broth. Others are "shakes" or drinks. Just take care to find one that is low in sugar (fewer than 4 grams) and actually high in protein (more than 20 grams) in each serving.

CANCER AND SUPPLEMENTS: CAUTION!

As we have alluded to throughout this chapter, it is not uncommon for people with cancer to use dietary supplements during and after cancer treatment—as many 30 percent during treatment and 80 percent at some point after treatment is over. The studies that have looked at supplement use in cancer patients have not been designed to unequivocally prove a relationship between supplements and the outcome of treatments, either good or bad, but the scientific data that we do have is not promising. For example, one study that looked at supplement use among more than a thousand women with breast cancer found that taking antioxidant supplements, which includes common vitamins like A, C, and E, before and during treatment actually increased the risk of a woman's cancer coming back and, to a lesser extent, their risk of dying. Despite how common supplement use is among people with cancer, more than two-thirds of doctors do not know whether their patients are taking supplements.

The scientific evidence for how supplements might interact with cancer treatments is relatively scant, but as Dr. Thomson pointed out to me, the medical community has not even clearly established the recommended daily amounts (RDAs) of common minerals and vitamins for people with cancer, let alone which ones you might want to supplement during treatment. As a result, many oncologists are wary of them. For example, some dietary supplements can cause severe reactions when taken during radiation treatment. If you are getting chemotherapy and you take certain supplements, you may be at higher risk of drug interactions; certain supplements may also interfere with your body's natural metabolic processes, causing cancer medicines to stay in your body for shorter or longer amounts of time than they should. There is also a concern that antioxidants might interfere with the way that treatments actually kill cancer cells.

Thus taken as a whole, it is best to strive for balance. "If you get too little or too much of almost any nutrient, you will have physiological responses that are going to reduce the efficacy of treatments and the outcome after cancer," Dr. Thomson told me.

When thinking about balance, we can again take vitamin C as an example, which has an RDA of 75 to 90 milligrams per day. An orange has about 50 milligrams of vitamin C. One or two oranges a day would put you right in the sweet spot—neither too much nor too little. By comparison, an average vitamin C supplement at your local pharmacy might have 500 or 1,000 milligrams per pill. That's the equivalent of eating ten to twenty oranges. Some powdered formulations have 4,000 milligrams per serving—the equivalent of forty oranges.

If your doctor prescribes a dietary supplement for a specific nutrient deficiency, which is not uncommon during cancer treatment, then by all means you should take it as prescribed. But taking supplements that have unnatural amounts of vitamins or minerals in them is not a balanced approach to nutrition and may even be causing harm. If you do decide to take supplements or multivitamins during treatment, be sure to tell your nurses and physicians.

PRACTICAL NUTRITION TIPS

To outline the general framework for nutrition during cancer treatment and afterward as a survivor: Strive to eat more fruits, vegetables, and protein and look at your diet as a pattern over the course of weeks rather than a snapshot on a particular day. But how exactly do you do this, given that healthy eating is just one of many priorities during cancer treatment? Here are some practical tips that can help.

Enjoy food. Don't get so scripted with your diet that it causes you anxiety. The idea is to take a long view and tip the balance toward smarter, healthier choices. Try not to get hung up on "bad diet days" or obsess over the food choices you make.

Remember that you are not going to be doing this forever. Try to make the best effort you can right now knowing that you will eventually be through cancer treatment. This is especially true if your treatments are interfering with your ability to eat or enjoy food. Eating during cancer treatment can seem like work, especially if you are experiencing some of the treatment side effects we discuss later in this chapter, but remember that it is important to get adequate nutrition during this window of time so that you can get through your treatments successfully and move on.

Enlist your friends and family. This begins by identifying the right person. For many of us, there is already a "food reward person" in our lives—this is the one who bakes cookies or brings pastries to every gathering. Engage this person to direct their energy in a positive way—instead of baked goods, you can tell them how incredibly helpful it would be to receive a healthy frozen meal that you can bake or warm up on particularly draining days. You can also ask them to go grocery shopping for you if you are too tired or busy. If you have found the right person, they will be delighted—this is the person in your life who wants to help with food.

Use a meal delivery service. Nutritionists are seeing more and more cancer patients use meal delivery services to supplement home cooking, especially during periods of heavy fatigue. There are now dozens of these services and most ship to every zip code in the United States. Likewise, use ready-made foods like take-out or frozen dinners if you are very fatigued or to prevent nausea during cooking, if this is a problem.

Stay hydrated. It is important to stay hydrated during cancer treatment. Try to pay attention to your fluid intake. Basic water is fantastic, of course, but you can also think about other less obvious options like soup broth, consommé, milk and milkshakes, and fruit and vegetable juices. You can even incorporate it into dessert by eating Jell-O, ice pops and Popsicles, or frozen yogurt, sorbet, or ice cream.

Start in the produce section. When grocery shopping, start in the produce section and fill up your cart as much as possible with fruits and vegetables of different colors and varieties.

Try new foods. Once a week, try a new fruit or vegetable. It's amazing how many people have only had a half dozen varieties of fruits, or a half dozen kinds of vegetables, in their entire life.

Simplify your shopping list. This is probably not the time for elaborate meal planning, at least not regularly. At the grocery store, rather than shop for complicated recipes, it can be helpful to think more simply: Pick a vegetable, a fruit, a protein, and a grain—that's one meal. The point is this: You don't need to be making a lot of decisions around food because you're probably already tired of making decisions.

Meal replacements. These can be especially helpful if you are having a hard time meeting the recommended amount of daily protein. As one example, Ensure Max Protein has 30 grams of protein per drink, with just 1 gram of sugar.

Keep your weight stable. While weight loss is very common before and during cancer treatment, weight gain is also quite common. For example, some people with cancer find themselves "stress eating," often carbohydrates late at night, during periods of higher anxiety. If you are not actively trying to increase your food intake due to a side effect of treatment, like nausea or a sore mouth, then try to keep your weight stable during treatment with commonsense approaches like eating a lot of fruits and vegetables and limiting your fat intake by cooking with low-fat methods like steaming and grilling.

If you are nauseous, stay away from favorites. If you are vomiting frequently, abstain from your favorite foods for a time. If you love spaghetti, but you are nauseated and throw it up, you may never want to eat it again. This can become symbolic as well. When treatment is finally over, you can throw out those meal replacements you never want to see again and instead return to your cherished favorites—letting go of foods and meals that you associate with cancer treatment can be a powerful and symbolic milestone on your journey.

Be systematic. Certain cancers and their treatments can cause severe gastrointestinal problems like bloating. If you are experiencing side effects like bloating, nausea, and vomiting, test foods that are commonly problematic by eliminating them from your diet one at a time to see if that helps.

If you've never really cooked before, try it. Some people really get energized by the self-efficacy, creativity, and confidence they feel when they realize they can cook.

Grow your own food. Cancer diagnoses are very often periods of deep self-reflection. Tending to something, whether it be a basil plant on your windowsill, a tomato plant in a pot on your patio, or a full-on vegetable garden, will cultivate and deepen that sense of self-reflection and connect you to the food you are eating.

Apply for assistance programs. If you are eligible, especially if you live alone or cannot shop for food or make meals, you may qualify for a food assistance program like God's Love We Deliver or Meals on Wheels. You can contact them directly online or ask your oncologist if there is a social worker or patient navigator at your cancer center who can help you apply.

SYMPTOM STRATEGIES

Beyond the basics outlined above, dietary needs during cancer treatment are often highly individualized. Cancer and cancer treatments can have many different effects on your ability to get adequate nutrition. Some of these are direct effects, like surgery or radiation to the gastrointestinal tract, which can interfere with your ability to chew, swallow, or digest foods. Others are so-called indirect effects, meaning that treatment—often systemic ones like chemotherapy—affect your body's metabolism.

Some of the most common side effects include a diminished appetite, nausea and vomiting, abdominal pain, diarrhea, and constipation. A few of these, like nausea, can occur with any of the routine cancer treatments. Others, like dry mouth or difficulty swallowing, tend to be associated with chemotherapy or with radiation specifically to the head and neck regions.

If you are experiencing any of these specific issues, be sure to bring them up with your oncologist. They may refer you to specialized nutrition counseling or prescribe medications that can help improve your symptoms. With nutrition during treatment, you want to get ahead of any problems—it is much easier to prevent nutrition problems during cancer treatment than it is to correct them.

Here are a few of the most common nutrition-related side effects and some strategies to help with them. For more information, the National Cancer Institute has published a number of resources for patients on nutrition during cancer care, which can be found online; Memorial Sloan Kettering Cancer Center, a highly regarded cancer center in New York City, also has resources on nutrition and diet during cancer treatment, including lists of recipes for cancer patients, on their website.

Loss of appetite and weight loss

- When you sit down for a meal, eat your protein first when your appetite is strongest.

- Add extra protein and calories to food by cooking with protein-fortified milk or using meal replacement drinks like Ensure in place of milk in your cereal.

- Eat your largest meal whenever you are hungriest, regardless of whether it is breakfast, lunch, or dinner.

- Move and be active to stimulate your appetite.

- Consider blending foods to make easier-to-consume nutrient-dense drinks.

Constipation

- Drink plenty of fluids each day.

- Eat more fiber in your diet.

- Stay active, including taking regular walks.

- Ask your doctor about taking fiber supplements or using laxatives or stool softeners.

- If you are developing gas, eliminate these commonly problematic foods one at a time to see if it helps: broccoli, cabbage, cauliflower, and beans.

Diarrhea

- Drink plenty of fluids, including water and sports drinks, to replace fluid lost from diarrhea.

- Eat foods and drink liquids high in sodium and potassium, like bouillon or broth, bananas, and potatoes, to replenish these key nutrients.

- Eat low-fiber foods.

- Avoid high-fiber and high-sugar foods, very hot or very cold drinks, greasy and fried foods, foods that cause gas (see constipation section above), milk, alcohol, spicy foods, caffeinated drinks, and sugar-free drinks sweetened with xylitol or sorbitol.

Dry mouth

- Sip water throughout the day.

- Eat and drink sweet or tart foods, like lemonade, to make more saliva.

- Chew gum or suck hard candy, ice pops, or ice chips.

- Eat foods that are easy to swallow, like noodles, casseroles, stews, and soups.

- Avoid those that can hurt your mouth, like spicy, hard, or crunchy foods.

- Use lip balm.

- Rinse your mouth every couple of hours, but avoid using mouthwash with alcohol.

- Talk with your doctor about artificial saliva or other prescription products that can help moisten your throat and mouth.

Nausea and vomiting

- Eat bland, soft, easy-to-digest foods.

- Eat dry foods, like crackers and toast, and foods that are easy on your stomach, like plain yogurt and clear broth.

- Avoid strong food and drink smells and don't eat in rooms that have strong cooking smells.

- Sit up for the first hour after eating.

- Rinse your mouth before and after eating.

- Eat smaller meals throughout the day rather than three large meals.

- Try not to skip meals—counterintuitively, having an empty stomach can make nausea worse.

- Only sip or drink small amounts during meals to avoid feeling bloated.

- Eat a few dry foods, like toast or crackers, before you go to bed if you are waking up nauseous. Or leave them by your bedside and eat them first thing in the morning before getting out of bed.

- Talk with your doctor about anti-nausea medications.

Sore mouth

- Choose easy-to-eat foods like milkshakes, scrambled eggs, and yogurt.

- Cook foods until they are soft and tender.

- Blend or purée foods to make their consistency easier to eat.

- Drink with a straw to avoid painful parts of your mouth.

- Avoid hot foods.

- Suck on ice chips or ice pops to numb and soothe your mouth.

- Avoid acidic foods like citrus and tomatoes, as well as spicy and crunchy foods.

- Rinse your mouth throughout the day with a mixture of ¼ teaspoon baking soda, ⅛ teaspoon salt, and 1 cup warm water.

- Check your mouth daily for sores, white patches, or puffy and red areas.

- Avoid anything that can hurt or burn your mouth, such as alcoholic drinks, mouthwashes with alcohol, or toothpicks and other sharp objects.

Taste changes

- Maintain good oral hygiene.

- Use plastic utensils and avoid drinking from metal containers if foods taste "metallic" to you.

- Substitute poultry, fish, or eggs for red meat or substitute meat with plant-based, non-meat proteins.

- Add spices or sauces to foods.

- Add something sweet, like applesauce or jelly, to meat.

- Use lemon drops, gum, or mints if you have a metallic taste in your mouth. There are also special mouthwashes that can help.

Remember, like exercise and sleep, good nutrition directly supports your ability to withstand cancer treatments and increases your chances of having a good outcome. That said, there is no magic diet or antioxidant supplement with "cancer-fighting" properties. Throughout treatment, the goal is to develop a pattern of eating more fruits and vegetables and making sure you get enough protein, which is critical for your body during this time. Use the log described elsewhere in the book to record and track your protein intake as a way of ensuring you prioritize it.

CAREGIVERS

hances are, you were just handed this book by someone you love and that someone has had a diagnosis of cancer. This chapter is for you, the caregiver. You play a vital role in the well-being of your loved one. Further, you are going through the cancer journey yourself, so there are reasons to focus on you as well.

This chapter is divided into two sections. Part one is on taking care of the patient. Part two is on taking care of the caregiver.

TAKING CARE OF THE PATIENT

When my wife, Sara, was diagnosed with cancer, I had recently taken a job 90 miles west of where we lived. I had an apartment where I stayed during the week and I came home on the weekends, which I had been doing for several months. It was not possible for me to stop working at my new job, but I did work remotely more than usual during her treatment. Sara and I both are blessed to see our jobs more as a vocation than as "work." We are both passionate about what we do and neither of us wanted this cancer diagnosis to derail our professional mission.

That was a lovely idea, but then reality hit when she had surgery. Sara's surgery was on a bright fall morning in November. I had thought there would be more family support, but on the day of surgery it became clear: I. Was. It. It was going to be me caring for Sara more than anyone else. I panicked because (as I mentioned) I really love my work, and, oh by the way, I have two sons to whom I am quite devoted. The post-surgical care was much more complex than Sara and I had understood beforehand. And then there would be several months of combined chemotherapy and radiation. I knew I had to be there for her, but I had no idea how I was going to get it done without having to take a leave of absence from work.

I spoke with Rose Sturgeon, wife of a head and neck cancer survivor, for advice. What she told me was very simple but very helpful, and I will share it with you: If someone offers to help, say yes. This journey is going to be hard and it is going to last longer than you think it will, so ask for and accept help.

I then heard about the website www.lotsahelpinghands.com. It's a care calendar website that allows you to get the word out via email to anyone in your life who might be willing to drive to an appointment, make dinner, walk the dog, do the laundry, clean the house, sit the kids, do some shopping, or any other task that would make it easier for you to care for yourself and your loved one. I set up our account on the website and sent an email to family, friends, coworkers, and acquaintances. The website made it easy to email reminders, as well as to send out general updates about Sara's condition. It is well designed, easy to use, and I highly recommend it. When I sent out the request for help, I cast the net wide, hoping to get a little bit of help. I was so impressed with the generosity of this network of people. My son, who was on a break from college, moved in with Sara during her chemo and radiation treatments so that she would not be alone on nights when I was away at work. A neighbor we did not know particularly well drove Sara to appointments more times than I can count and made numerous dinners. Sara's friends came through in ways that helped me see how very loved she was by others. Sara's aunt and sister each flew from California to spend a week caring for her.

Having lived through this, I'll impart a bit of advice: Don't waste emotional energy wondering why some folks don't do more. Be grateful for the folks who come through for you. You are likely to be surprised by who comes through and who doesn't. Notice it and move on. I wish someone had told me this. I hope it is helpful to you.

When it comes to supporting your patient with regard to the material in this book, you have four jobs.

Take charge of the daily log. You should be in charge of the log. Make it yourself, or download it from www.movingthroughcancer.com, and keep track of your loved one's treatment symptoms, daily sleep, eating, moving (aerobic exercise), and lifting (strength training).

There is so much about caregiving that feels frustrating, like having your hands tied behind your back. Chemotherapy drips into the arm of the one you love and you watch, week after week, as their mouth sores develop, fatigue progresses, and/or they lose feeling in their hands and feet. So often you have to watch and support but feel you can do nothing. However, this is a place where you get to be in charge. Make that log! Keep track of it. The information in that log will be so helpful for doctors, surgeons, and nurses to know how your patient is tolerating treatment. By noting when exercise is done and when it is too hard to do, you will start to notice patterns. And you will likely know when something is wrong before the clinicians do. The log will be useful—keep the log.

Exercise with your patient. The second job you have is doing all of the activities assigned in this book alongside your loved one. You should be doing all the walking, biking, jogging, dancing, and lifting—repetition for repetition, step for step—as well. Exercise studies have shown that your loved one will be much more motivated to follow through on their exercise plan if they have a partner working out alongside them. You will learn much more about how they are feeling and it is a positive activity for the two of you to do together at a time when you may feel all you talk about is cancer.

Follow the advice regarding protein intake and sleep. The only things you don't need to do for yourself are the logging activities. Otherwise, follow the sleep hygiene rules and all of the exercises prescribed. It is common for caregivers to gain weight (I gained 20 pounds). This will attenuate that weight gain.

Delegate, with impunity. Be willing to delegate more than might be comfortable. Your job is to be sure that there are clothes to wear, not to supervise the doing of the laundry. That said, you will come to know quickly who can be counted on and who cannot. At the beginning, until you know, consider having someone on "standby" in case someone else flakes out. I enacted a "one strike, you're out" rule: If someone said they would make dinner and did not, we took them off the calendar for the remainder of the time we needed help. The last thing you need to be doing is wondering whether someone will come through "this time." You have bigger fish to fry. Let that stuff go.

TAKING CARE OF THE CAREGIVER

Why are we focusing on you, the caregiver, when you are not the one with cancer? Well, you matter. You are going through something too. But if that isn't enough for you, know this: Research shows that caregiver well-being impacts quality of cancer care. Some of these effects are direct. When the caregiver feels depressed, overwhelmed, or distracted, it stands to reason that caregiving tasks will be done with less competence. But there is even some suggestion that if caregivers are depressed or rate their own health poorly, patients may be more likely to be rehospitalized or to rate their own health more poorly.

The National Academy of Medicine issues reports on the most important topics in health care with expert panels of clinicians and researchers. One such report, published in 2013, was called "Delivering High-Quality Cancer Care: Charting a New Course for a System in Crisis." It outlines how informed, active, and participatory caregivers (and patients) help improve health care outcomes. Caregivers are crucial in this respect—you understand what is happening to the patient as well as, if not better than, anybody. You can attend medical appointments and assist the patient in clearly explaining symptoms. You can help make sure that the patient understands what the medical professionals are communicating. Research has shown that two people listening to a doctor together come away with a better recall of what a doctor says than one person alone. You can take notes or just provide a second set of ears. You can also help by coordinating appointments and insurance issues. Sometimes these issues get complex.

Finally, you may be called upon to help make decisions along the way. Your patient may need to decide between two or more courses of action. If you are actively participating in the process, you can help the patient weigh the options and gather the information needed to decide. All of this means you need to be taking care of yourself. Let me tell you a bit about how I did all this, in part as a cautionary tale.

MY STORY

Sara was diagnosed on Tuesday, October 11, 2016. The diagnosis was a shock, given her age and relatively good health. She had been complaining of "something in my nostril" for months and seeking an appropriate diagnosis. Three months before her diagnosis, an ear, nose, and throat doctor told her "there's nothing wrong with your nose" after she revealed to him that she was obsessed with noses and convinced something was wrong with hers.

When she was finally diagnosed with an aggressive squamous cell carcinoma in her nostril, we were both shocked and upset at the diagnosis and so overwhelmed that we basically went from appointment to appointment asking questions and ignoring the rest of our lives for the month between diagnosis and surgery. Initially, we were in complete disbelief. My mother had had a squamous cell skin cancer removed from her nose decades earlier and I mistakenly thought we were dealing with something similarly benign. It wasn't until an appointment with the whole team (medical, radiation, surgical oncology, reconstructive surgery, nursing, social worker) that we realized we were dealing with something much more serious. I can still recall thinking at the time that having all those people in the room for this small thing in Sara's nose was overkill. And then Sara started crying and the energy in the room kind of "broke."

We all came to the same place: This was serious. I can still remember exactly where I was, what chair I was sitting in, and who was in the room the moment I first wondered whether the cancer would take Sara's life. Time stopped.

To say that cancer caregiving is hard is an understatement. Perhaps if I place it in context of other difficulties in my life that might help. I would say it is as hard as my divorce from my children's father, but not as hard as the death of my parents. Another way of expressing it is to say that it is overwhelming. Suddenly, in the midst of my busy life, I was adding dozens of appointments, a great deal of uncertainty, and a serious disfigurement of my partner's face into the mix. That just about says it.

I was overwhelmed over and over and over again. But in the same way that a parent with a teething infant just keeps walking the floor and holding their baby, you just keep going. You stop thinking about it. But it takes a toll. For me, I stopped exercising, drank a glass of wine every night (too much), and slept poorly. I wish you better coping than I managed for myself.

Sara's surgery was particularly overwhelming. She was in the hospital for five days following her rhinectomy and initial forehead flap reconstruction. By day two, it became clear that caring for her wound at home was going to be extensive. They said they would teach me and then ran through the instructions at lightning pace. I felt totally underprepared for what I was being asked to do for Sara. Luckily, I was able to convince her sister Sandy, a wound care nurse, to visit for a week and do the early wound care. Sandy was the one who taught me, carefully, expertly, how to care for the extensive skin grafts Sara had received. Without that help, I think there would have been less sleep and more worry, and I wonder whether she would have healed as well as she did.

I was still living in two places and commuting 90 miles to work during this period. After the surgery, Sara took four months off of work to recover and get through her chemotherapy and radiation. I set up an army of supporters to make her dinner, visit, stay with her, run errands, and otherwise ensure she was OK during the days that I had to be away. And I worked from home a lot too.

One of my greatest regrets from that period is that I did not take a more active role in making sure that Sara was getting proper nutrition, exercise, and sleep, and that I was getting these things too.

When it came time for the combined chemo and radiation, the big task was coordinating the small army of people who came out of the woodwork to help. There was always a backup person, in case someone could not do the task they agreed to do. I may not have been there for every chemo visit, but I was the orchestra conductor ensuring that someone Sara knew and liked was there for every single appointment, every meal, and every evening. As I mentioned, my son Mack moved into the house with Sara during this time, so that there was never a night she was alone if I had to be away at work. I think the bond formed between Mack and Sara as a result of this time will be something they treasure forever.

Several things surprised me along the way. One was the sheer volume of time demanded for all of the appointments. I went to many of them. I would never describe myself as "patient." (When I read this sentence to my wife she laughed out loud.) It was incredibly frustrating how much time was spent waiting for doctors and nurses to do whatever was next in a given appointment. This has been described by some in the field of oncology as the "toxicity of time." The one upside to this was that Sara and I discovered our mutual enjoyment of HGTV, which seems to be the generic channel on in all cancer treatment waiting rooms. We have carried this forward since Sara's treatment ended.

Sara's extreme disfigurement was a unique aspect of her cancer journey and one that she still lives with (to a lesser extent now, but it's still an issue). Sara made peace with her new face long before I did. At one point, she said she was OK with how she looked and did not care what anyone else thought or felt. It took me two years to talk to her about how I felt about the way surgery had changed her. It is a natural human response to disfigurement to be repulsed, to feel revulsion. And I did feel this, for many months. My attraction to Sara declined significantly, given the change in her appearance. And based on what she said to me, she did not seem to care. I felt very guilty about my feelings, because I was walking around with a normal face. Who was I to feel ANYTHING but sympathy and kindness when Sara was the one with the missing nose and the scarred, disfigured face?

The truth is that it is normal to feel revulsion in the face of disfigurement. But it was not until I admitted those feelings, not just to myself but also to Sara, that I could start to move past them. It was a very difficult set of conversations and the relationship felt rocky for a while. But today I actually prefer Sara's face without her prosthetic nose. This is, in part, because the glue smells bad, but mostly it's because all I really see when I look at Sara are her eyes and her smile. It has taken me time to get here, but I do really feel like I am as attracted to Sara now as I was when I first met her. Perhaps the universal aspect of this experience, across all cancer caregivers, is that caregivers will have their own feelings about their patient's cancer, and those feelings are valid and need to be handled with the same kindness and attention as the feelings of the cancer patient.

Another surprise was that Sara wasn't "better" right after treatment. In retrospect, that sounds like an unreasonable expectation. But after four months of cancer treatments, when she rang that bell with gusto, we were fully prepared for her to be "better." When she felt worse a week or two later, we were so frustrated when her doctors told us this was to be expected. Had they mentioned this and we missed it? Had they assumed we knew? We'll never know. We certainly believe in the good intentions of all the clinicians who treated Sara, but this was one of many instances when we were surprised by something and felt the clinicians had not adequately prepared us. This is a common experience among cancer patients and their caregivers. As such, you should expect the unexpected. Be ready to roll with what comes.

I also wish that Sara's doctors had made it clear that when they told us what was coming (first A, then B, then C) they were generally not giving us the full story. In many instances, the truth may be that after A, new information is learned that may require the addition of Q to the plan, and after Q, there may be yet another change of plans. In Sara's case, the story line at the beginning was that Sara would not need chemotherapy; the plan was surgery and radiation. On the day after Thanksgiving, her surgeon called and said that certain aspects of the surgery had not gone to plan and that they did not get clear margins (meaning the entire tumor had not been removed). A week later, we were told that the pathologist was concerned about how aggressive the cancer appeared to be on the microscope. With these factors taken together, it was now recommended that she get chemotherapy as well.

Similar pivots happened throughout the reconstruction process as well. It would be easy to feel lied to by the clinicians, but the truth is, they were giving us the best possible information they had every time they spoke with us. And it could be that if they had told us that there was a possibility of unclear margins and an aggressive tumor type, it would have worried us more than they thought was necessary. Another viewpoint is that they withheld information that we could have used to help make better decisions. I'll let you decide.

Another major issue that I have dealt with as a caregiver, and still do, is the distance created between Sara and me by my fear of her cancer recurrence or possible death. This is an ongoing issue. Sara's cancer is a particularly aggressive one, with a 65 percent likelihood of returning within five years. While writing this book, Sara is now four years out from the end of her cancer treatment, close to that magical five-year mark many consider to be a threshold signifying a lower risk of cancer recurrence. (Whether that is true or not in Sara's case is unknown, given how rare the cancer is.) But to this day, I continue to wrestle with this issue. It seems to run something like this: 1) I get crabby with Sara, 2) I pull away, 3) she notices and gets upset, 4) I don't understand what's happening, nor does she, 5) I remember that I'm afraid of her recurrence risk. I feel afraid for a bit, and we move on. Until the next round.

Ultimately, my work, my health, my relationship, and my weight were all adversely affected by Sara's cancer. I'm not sure that I want to say that I did anything wrong, per se, but there were some things I could have done better.

Here's what I wish for you:

1. Do all the exercises with your loved one. As noted in the first section, it will give you something positive to focus on, something within your control.

2. Focus on getting high-quality sleep.

3. Follow the dietary recommendations in chapter 14.

4. Avoid alcohol and other inebriants. These are not going to help when you need to be rested and clearheaded for the many decisions and tasks that caring for someone with cancer demands.

5. Consider working with a psychology professional. A good therapist can be a great neutral listener to hear what is gross, creepy, difficult, wearisome, and otherwise unpleasant about what you are doing, seeing, and experiencing.

6. If you get to the other side of the experience and you are still breathing, count it as a win. This is a hard thing to do. If you do nothing else, pat yourself on the back for just surviving it. I do.

16

ATHLETES

I n each of the preceding chapters, the recommendations we have
made are based on a level of scientific evidence on which I would
stake my professional reputation as an exercise oncology researcher.

This chapter is different. The truth is that there are simply not
enough high-level athletes undergoing cancer treatment to run the kinds
of scientific trials we have talked about in previous chapters. This is, at
least in part, because of the relationship between regular physical activity and the prevention of multiple common types of cancer, including
breast, colon, endometrial, kidney, bladder, esophageal, and stomach
cancers. This evidence was highlighted in the recent American College of
Sports Medicine Roundtable guidelines for cancer prevention and control, as well as the recent US Department of Health and Human Services
Physical Activity Guidelines Advisory Committee.

However, the fact that athletes develop cancer is evidence that exercise is not a foolproof preventive for cancer. The opposite corollary is that
not everyone who smokes gets cancer, but it is definitely a risk. We are
quite sure that people who are more active are less likely to develop cancer. But when they do, they undoubtedly want to know what they should
and should not do in order to get the best possible cancer outcome.

So what do we know? Sigh. The answer is largely anecdotal.

As mentioned in chapter 3, to really know something with scientific certainty, we need what my mentor Dr. Henry Blackburn called the "three beauties": evidence from each of the major types of medical studies—basic science studies, often using animals or even single cells; clinical studies assessing a specific intervention in dozens or hundreds of patients; and epidemiologic studies that look at patterns of behavior, like exercising, across thousands of people. When all of these different kinds of studies provide results that point in the same direction, we can really be confident about a cause-and-effect relationship.

But the pool of people who really want to push themselves physically during cancer treatment is relatively small. And cancer researchers focus their efforts, very appropriately, on helping as many cancer patients as they can. Trials focused on athletic cancer patients and survivors would benefit few.

So at the moment we do not have these "three beauties." We may never have them. But however small, this group—those who want to train hard during and after cancer treatment—is growing. And it includes people who not only want to get back to where they were before cancer, but to exceed it and set personal bests when cancer treatment is behind them.

So, a caveat: We do not have firm scientific data on how cancer treatment and high-level exercise training interact. Instead, we have a list of lessons learned from athletes ranging from recreational marathoners to US track and field champions, from college lacrosse players to Olympic gold medalists. These include people who run 5Ks in the middle of their radiation treatments to those who finish Ironman triathlons in between chemotherapy cycles. They are proof that it is possible to train hard and achieve incredible accomplishments despite cancer treatment.

Their stories follow. But here are the most important points for training hard during and after cancer treatment, taken from their experience.

You can likely do more than you think you can. Cancer treatment will invariably decondition your body. That said, the body is capable of being trained during treatment, and if you enter treatment in good shape, you can do incredible things during treatment.

Set realistic goals. This is highly personal and based on both your previous training levels and your response to treatment. You will almost certainly not be setting personal bests in the months during cancer treatment. Knowing that, try to assess what would be a meaningful goal to achieve, something that excites and motivates you but is not unreasonable given all of the physical and other demands on your life at this time.

Listen to your body. This is the one point that every high-level athlete interviewed for this book agreed on. You know best what your body is telling you and if it is saying that it needs time to rest and heal, give it that time. Finishing your cancer treatment successfully will always be the most important goal. Toward this goal, we strongly recommend that you adopt the habit of logging your symptoms and getting adequate protein intake, sleep, and aerobic and resistance exercise daily. See chapter 2 for instructions on logging.

Don't push yourself too hard too early. The tissues of your nervous and musculoskeletal systems will respond to treatment in different ways. Especially after surgery, parts of your body may feel ready to get back to heavy lifting or vigorous training right away, while others need a more gradual reintroduction. Err on the side of caution. If a surgical wound gets infected or you tear a ligament, it will set you back weeks, if not months. And, unfortunately, this is really common among athletes who go through cancer treatment.

Change your focus. As you will read on the following pages, some athletes achieve lifelong dreams after a cancer diagnosis, whether that is qualifying for the Boston Marathon, finishing an Ironman triathlon, or even becoming a US champion in their sport. That said, to a person, they agreed that living through cancer changed the focus of their efforts. Personal best performances became less important; simply enjoying the ability to get outside and feel healthy became much more central. Whereas the focus of their training pre-cancer was often self-centered, after treatment they looked outward, using exercise as a way to connect with family or their community or, quite often, to raise money for worthy causes.

KIKKAN RANDALL:
HAVE THE CONFIDENCE THAT YOU CAN KEEP DOING WHAT YOU ARE USED TO DOING

We first met Kikkan Randall in chapter 4, where she talked about the level of fatigue that even Olympic athletes feel during chemotherapy. Though that was a low point for her during treatment, it was the exception, not the rule. In fact, when Kikkan was diagnosed with breast cancer she was three months out from her gold medal–winning performance at the 2018 Winter Olympics and in the best shape of her career as the most decorated cross-country skier—man or woman—in US history. And though she recognized that breast cancer treatment was naturally going to alter her post-Olympic exercise goals, she had no plan to stop them completely.

"When I got the diagnosis, literally my first reaction was, 'I'm just going to keep doing what I can,'" Kikkan told me.

Kikkan took the same approach she did in the months leading up to the birth of her son. "It was actually very similar to what I went through when I was pregnant with my son, in that there's not a lot of guidelines out there telling you what you can or cannot do," Kikkan said. "During my pregnancy, I was pleasantly surprised by how much I was able to do. I just made the rule that I would follow my body. If I was feeling good, I would do what I had planned. And if not, I was always able to back down. So I went into my cancer treatment with the same kind of philosophy—I am going to keep doing what I love to do and just make sure I follow my body, knowing that I need to rest and recover through it as well."

Practically speaking, this meant tailoring her workouts to her three-week chemotherapy cycles, just as we recommended in chapter 7. The first week or week and a half after a treatment, when she felt the worst, her daily exercise might consist of a very slow 30-minute jog or an easy spin on the bicycle. During the second week, she would gradually ramp up the intensity, and by week three, when she was feeling strong again, she was incorporating interval training into her aerobic exercise sessions and doing at least two strength-training sessions per week in the gym.

However, like most people getting chemotherapy, her fatigue and other side effects were cumulative over the course of her treatment. By the last two or three rounds of treatment, she found she was not bouncing back quite as quickly by the end of her second week. So for the last month and a half of treatment, she abandoned her interval training and anything else particularly intense, though she continued to do about an hour of exercise at some level every day. She also took longer breaks between her lifts during strength-training sessions. Even though Kikkan had spent her entire life following training plans, her approach during chemotherapy was to "try not to have too much of a set idea of what I was going to do exactly." This meant backing down or "calling it early" if she didn't feel good.

That said, she never stopped training—it was essential to how she saw herself and her life outside cancer treatment. "To me, that was why exercise was so important—it helped me feel normal through this process. And it helped me stay true to my identity as an athlete."

Her advice: "Have the confidence that you can keep doing what you're used to doing. Listen to your body. You may not be able to do everything at the level you are used to through the whole treatment, but just keep building. That will make it easier to build back up when you are through the majority of treatment as well."

MEGAN HART:
BE AMBITIOUS, BUT NOT DANGEROUSLY SO

As she entered her junior year at Shippensburg University in Pennsylvania, Megan Hart had high athletic ambitions: The Raiders lacrosse team, where she was a forward, was looking to repeat as national champions. Inside the classroom, she was doing coursework in exercise science with the goal of eventually becoming a strength and conditioning coach.

Yet something was off. She was deeply fatigued and her joints ached to the point that she was having trouble walking. The trainers at Shippensburg implored her to figure out what was going on. Finally, a week into the school year she went home to rest. That weekend she ended up in the ER with a 105-degree fever and a white cell count near zero. Pediatric oncologists diagnosed her with acute lymphoblastic leukemia.

Megan, whom I met through the Adolescent and Young Adult Cancer Survivors support activities at the Penn State Cancer Institute, has an indefatigable spirit and a driven personality. She has also had a very difficult cancer journey. She was under active cancer treatment for two and half years, including a five-month hospitalization for a rare fungal infection. Her muscles had atrophied to the point that she essentially had to learn to walk again. However, true to form, by the end of her hospital stay she was playing field hockey in the hallways of the inpatient cancer unit, passing a hockey ball back and forth with a couple of nurses who had played in high school.

Back at home, she started with the goal of simply walking to the mailbox and back. Eventually, she started swimming in her grandmother's pool, and finally, running 2 miles through the hills near her parents' home in Juniata County, Pennsylvania.

Like many active people who undergo cancer treatment, Megan had a difficult time reconciling her "new normal" with the standout athlete she had been previously, the most valuable player on both her high school field hockey and track and field teams. "The hardest thing was that before, I always knew I could run a certain pace and lift a certain amount of weight, but it was the realization that I couldn't do that right now. That was the frustrating point—I felt, I could do this before, so why can't I do it now?"

Megan used her background in exercise science to develop a strength-training program that included high-repetition endurance-style lifting as well as strength-building types of lifts. On Tuesdays, Thursdays, and Saturdays, she would do either a longer-distance run or take a cycling class, eventually becoming a certified spinning instructor. Her hard work paid off: She was able to return to the lacrosse field in regular season competition. As her name was called over the PA system at Shippensburg University, everyone in the stands stood and cheered for the girl who had come back from cancer. "It was a very proud and humbling moment that, you know, I overcame everything that I've been through and then I've worked so hard to get to that specific point."

Unfortunately Megan pushed herself too hard. Shortly after her 2018 season, she tore her anterior cruciate ligament playing in an indoor field hockey league. "My problem was that I made a goal that was way too big for myself," Megan said.

I have unfortunately seen this many times, especially in younger, ambitious athletes with a background in heavy lifting. During cancer treatment, the body is deconditioned, and in particular there is a loss of muscle. The nervous system, however, can be far less affected. Put simply, if you were an Olympic lifter who could clean and jerk 200 pounds before cancer treatment, the neuromuscular circuits remain intact to perform this same movement after treatment. But the number and strength of muscle fibers required to perform a heavy lift like this may have deteriorated significantly. The combination, added on top of the desire to prove that you haven't "lost it" despite cancer treatment, can be dangerous. Every exercise scientist who has treated cancer patients for any amount of time has seen this happen.

"If you have a goal, strive to reach it, but don't be disappointed if you can't specifically reach that goal," Megan said of her experience. "Realize that it's OK to just take a break sometimes and just give your body the relaxation and the recovery that it needs."

SINDY HOOPER:
ANYTHING IS POSSIBLE

Shortly after Sindy Hooper first started treatment for pancreatic cancer, she told her husband, Jon, that she had made a decision: She was not going to cancel her plans to compete in the Ironman Canada triathlon later that year in Whistler, British Columbia. Jon, an anesthesiologist and intensive care doctor at the Ottawa Hospital and frequent medical director for local 5K races, was floored: "The first thought in my head was 'Jesus Christ.'"

If anyone had borne witness to Sindy's determination and grit, it was Jon. Sindy hadn't started doing triathlons until her late forties, but for much of her training Jon had been swimming, running, and biking right alongside his hard-charging wife.

But he also knew how difficult Sindy's treatment was going to be. The surgery to remove her tumor, known as a Whipple procedure, is among the most complex cancer surgeries done and involves removing the head of the pancreas, the first part of the small intestine, the gallbladder, and the bile duct, and then reconnecting the remaining gastrointestinal organs. She would then have eighteen rounds of IV chemotherapy, bisected by a month of radiation. And throughout it all, she was planning to train for one of the most difficult one-day sporting events in the world: a 2.4-mile (3.86-km) swim, a 112-mile (180.25-km) bicycle ride, and a marathon 26.22-mile (42.20-km) run, raced in that order. Astonishingly, she planned to complete the race during the very depths of her treatment—eight months into her nine-month treatment plan, when her side effects would likely have accumulated to their very worst.

"I said to my [surgeon], 'So do you think it might be possible for me to do the Ironman in August?' And he looked at me like I was crazy," Sindy said. "I described the distances and he was just shaking his head and said, 'I don't understand why a healthy person would want to do that, let alone somebody who's about to go through what you're about to go through.'"

Sindy is not the type to be dissuaded by a bit of disbelief. In her own words, she has "a huge type-A personality, I'm very competitive, and I can push myself pretty hard. And it was important for me to be able to take part in this event." Both her oncologist and her husband were worried that she was going to push herself to an unsafe place, so they set about making a plan.

The first was establishing that finishing treatment was by far more important than finishing the Ironman. "Sindy and I had an agreement that I would pull the plug on her if I thought she was overdoing it," Jon said. "We talked about it several times—that treatment was the number-one goal and the Ironman was second. If this started going off the rails, I was going to be brutally honest and she would have to listen to me. We had that conversation several times to make it abundantly clear because Sindy will go hard and she won't want to quit."

The second was taking a scientific approach to her training plan. Sindy trained at the Peak Centre for Human Performance in Ottawa, where her coach tested her blood lactate levels to understand how her body was responding to training during cancer treatment. Not surprisingly, previously modest efforts were now much more physically taxing. Her coach took all high-intensity training out of the program. He prescribed exclusively "zone 1" training, meaning that Sindy's heart rate during exercise should remain around 50 to 60 percent of her maximum heart rate and that, alternately, if she were using the breath test we've mentioned throughout this book, she should be able to speak easily in full sentences throughout her workouts. Instead of going out for an hour-long tempo run, as she would have done previously, Sindy was forced to walk briskly and only run the downhills if she felt well enough and her heart rate remained in zone 1.

The final part of the plan was to train for distance, not power or speed. Sindy went into her surgery in phenomenal shape, having completed an Ironman just five months prior. Despite being incredibly lean, she still lost more than 10 percent of her body weight after surgery, essentially all of it muscle. Though she did specific strength training throughout her nine months of treatment, her strength and power did not return.

"My power and intensity didn't really go up, but I was able to do my swimming, biking, and running for longer and longer periods of time," Sindy said. "That was very easy to see from the logs that I kept." (Note: Sindy clearly agrees that keeping a log is helpful.)

Even with these precautions, there were still moments when Sindy crossed the line. "There were a couple of instances where we were out on the bike and Jon had to pull the plug on me and say, 'No, you're stopping. You're done.' I was in tears, telling him, 'I don't want to stop. I have to do this.' But it was a good thing because I would've pushed myself. I would've fainted or passed out or crashed my bike."

On the whole, however, it was good for her. "Training for Ironman always made me feel better," Sindy said. "I could be sitting indoors on the couch, feeling nauseous and horrible, but I always felt better when I went outside. I got this reprieve from feeling like a cancer patient to feeling like somebody who was healthy. That was a huge part of it for me."

Training was going well and Sindy was hitting her targets, but nevertheless she was filled with uncertainty. "We were never really confident that I would actually be able to do the Ironman. I knew I could do the swim. And then we were going to do the first part of the bike course and then just take it from there."

The bigger concern was far more terrifying: Sindy was eight months out from her diagnosis. On average, just 20 percent of pancreatic cancer patients live to a year. She was fearing for her life.

In August, they went to Whistler for race day with a group of friends. Sindy finished the swim as planned. The bike ride, however, was contentious. Jon kept insisting that Sindy take breaks on the more difficult hills so that she didn't expend all of her energy too early. "She got pissed off at me a few times, saying, 'We're not going to make it.'" They finished the bike course with 15 minutes to spare before the cut-off time. And having preserved just enough energy, Sindy managed to finish the marathon run as well.

"The fact that I actually completed an Ironman was a miracle. We never expected that to happen," Sindy said. It was an incredible moment, demonstrating that anything is possible, even during the hardest moments of cancer treatment.

Since then, however, Sindy has had to reconcile her type-A, competitive personality with the limits of what her body can do post-cancer. "It's been seven and a half years since Ironman Canada, and it's been extremely frustrating because I have not been hitting my goals. I still feel like I'm training really hard, but I have not been able to get back to even close to where I was pre-cancer," Sindy said. "That's really frustrating because I keep pushing and thinking, 'It's going to come, it's going to come' and then it doesn't come. It's really upsetting and frustrating." The biggest difference that she's noticed is that her body is not predictable: "Before cancer, it was all amazing. Now it's all over the place. I can get some really great training days and I can get some really horrible training days."

Sindy remains competitive in her age group, but in these races pre-cancer she would have been on the podium. She is still faster than many of her friends and training partners, even younger ones, and she has qualified and raced the Boston Marathon since finishing treatment, an accomplishment considered to be a lifelong achievement for many distance runners, cancer or no cancer.

The disappointment has led to a shift in both her perspective and her goals: She now often runs to fundraise for charities. "Racing for me used to be very self-centered. I still love to race for the spirit of racing, but now it's so much bigger than that. I still try to qualify for the Boston Marathon and if I don't make it, I'm extremely disappointed, but there is also this silver lining that even though I didn't qualify for Boston, look at all the other stuff that I accomplished from it. It's not a different goal. It's just a broader goal," Sindy said. "And I'm lucky that I'm still here, that I'm still alive. Instead of worrying that I haven't qualified for [the Ironman World Championships in] Kona yet, I tell myself, 'Well, thank God, I'm still here eight years after this horrible cancer diagnosis.'"

JOHN MURRAY: THE GREAT RESET

John Murray was on the biggest and most exciting business trip of his life. He had created his dream job—setting up global NBA games—and was at the end of a forty-day business trip that included kicking off the International Basketball Federation World Cup tournament in China and meeting with a group of businessmen in Doha, Qatar, to discuss upcoming opportunities for the 2022 FIBA World Cup. Near the end of the trip, he took a detour to Ha Long Bay in Vietnam, a UNESCO World Heritage Site and one of the most beautiful places in the world, to travel with a friend. When he woke up from what he thought was a great nap, his friend told him that he had had a seizure.

Sped by boat to a Vietnamese hospital and eventually home to St. Paul, Minnesota, John underwent an MRI that revealed he had a tumor, an astrocytoma, the size of his hand lodged in his brain. Before surgery to remove it, his surgeons told him what they thought his life might look like post-surgery: They were hopeful that they could get 60 percent of the tumor out, but that he might be blind, lose some of his Chinese language skills, or not be able to run in the future. He went under the knife on

"Marathon Monday," the annual running of the Boston Marathon on the third Monday of April.

He awoke from the nine-hour surgery, which went better than expected, and was asked to perform a few simple cognitive tests, like sticking out his tongue and uttering a few phrases in Chinese. Once it was clear that he was OK—though still heavily drugged with anesthesia—John made a startling pronouncement to the surgical team: He too would run the Boston Marathon.

People are known to say many strange things in the hour or so after major surgeries, and this one ranks right up there—qualifying for the Boston Marathon is highly competitive and John still had to undergo radiation to his head as well as rounds of chemotherapy to kill the small amount of remaining tumor left in his brain. But having spent several years in China, John followed Lao Tzu's famous proverb: "The journey of a thousand miles begins with a single step."

In the years before his cancer diagnosis, John, a self-described "classic runner's-high guy," was building his international marketing business; running brought focus, meaning, and purpose to a lifestyle that was, quite literally, all over the place. He started running as a way to give structure to his life, and what began with half-mile and mile runs turned into 5Ks and 10Ks, and eventually marathons and a 50K.

Like so many endurance athletes who love the runner's high, the quest is always to go farther, faster. John was hitting his numbers, but his efforts had become all-consuming. "At a certain point I was accomplishing my goals, but having less and less fun," John said of that time.

Cancer treatment would become "the great reset" of John's running life. He was no longer concerned whether he ran 7:06 or 7:01 miles; if he got out of bed, down the driveway, and up the street, it was amazing. "The physical side had always been important to me, but the mental side totally shifted."

John cleared all of his running with his oncologists, and they had one major concern: If he dehydrated himself, he was at risk of a second seizure. So while they told him to be very careful, they also encouraged him, recognizing that he had a good understanding of himself and his body.

"During chemo, running was not the obstacle for me, it was the cure," John said. Before cancer, John refused even to take a Tylenol. So if treatment left him constipated, John took his typical approach to the problem: He drank a cup of coffee and went for a run. "I was able to pinpoint these side effects of the drugs and treatments and running was often the way for me to get through them."

His seizure risk also turned his running into a family affair. His father rode his bike alongside him, plying him with Gatorade. His younger sister, a physician's assistant, took up running and now accompanies John on 10-milers, admonishing him to slow down, stay hydrated, and take care of himself. "In order to look after me, she herself had to become a runner," John said. "So the doctors that I had were all very supportive because they learned of the kind of intense, close family support I had." (Aside: Caregivers, are you getting this? You are encouraged to exercise with your patient step by step, rep by rep.)

Word of John's goal to run the Boston Marathon eventually reached Eliud Kipchoge, the world record holder in the marathon whom many consider the greatest marathoner of the modern era. "I shared my story and he said, 'John, keep running, please keep running. Your mind can heal anything.'"

Through a series of connections, he was also granted acceptance to the Boston Marathon on behalf of the Boston College Campus School, raising money for their special education program.

The marathon was ultimately canceled because of COVID-19, but John ran his own "mini-Boston Marathon" of 22 miles on the third Monday in April 2020 nonetheless.

Much more importantly, his diagnosis and the experience of training through treatment has completely changed how he looks at running. One lesson is the importance of letting go of expectations. "Previously, I had these goals. But now, throughout this process, I have looked more deeply within myself and said, 'What am I capable of doing that will bring me happiness?' This entire journey for me has been about dropping a lot of those kinds of thoughts that I once had and enjoying every moment of every run that I'm on."

John is running 7-minute miles again. But his goals now revolve around a much different Taoist principle he's incorporated into his training: "You need to laugh out loud three times every day. And I've learned that if I'm not doing that, then I'm not running correctly. It could be a quarter-mile run or it could be a 30-mile run, but you'll hear me—I'm the guy that will laugh three times on every run."

GABE GRUNEWALD:
BRAVE LIKE GABE

When John Murray ventured out into his local Minneapolis–St. Paul community to meet other runners post-cancer, the first organized run he went to in 2019 was in honor of a local hero: Gabe Grunewald. It was a memorial run; Gabe had recently passed from complications after a decade-long battle with a rare cancer, adenoid cystic carcinoma. But in her life as an athlete and cancer advocate, she embodied the very best principles of staying active despite a life-changing health diagnosis.

I had the immense honor of meeting Gabe and speaking with her about what she learned as an elite athlete fighting metastatic cancer before she passed away in 2019. Gabe's achievements as an athlete stand on their own; that she accomplished them while also fighting cancer make them truly remarkable.

A year after being diagnosed with cancer while in college, Gabe turned professional as a middle-distance runner in 2010, signing a contract with Brooks Sports. That year she also received a second cancer diagnosis, this one in her thyroid.

Despite this, a year later Gabe placed third nationally in the mile run both indoors and outdoors. In 2012, she was fourth in the 1500 meters at the US Olympic Trials, missing the Olympic team by one place. Two years later she would win the USA Championship title in the indoor 3000 meters. During this time, she also ran a 4:01.48 in the outdoor 1500 meters, making her the eleventh-fastest performer in US history.

These achievements made her message clear: Never give up hope. "I've actually heard from a lot of people who are trying to get back out there. They might be slower, and maybe they're not running their personal best, but they might be in a year or two," Gabe told me. "I tell them that as a two-time cancer survivor, I ran faster than I ever did in my life. You can be faster and you can do better after cancer. It is possible. Your potential might not be as low as you thought it was as a cancer survivor. You really can do a lot."

From a training perspective, Gabe emphasized the importance of setting meaningful, but realistic, goals. When I last spoke to her, for example, she was trying to break a 4:40 mile. Her "previous self" could run a 4:20 mile without too much of a problem, so even though it wasn't exciting to her from the standpoint of setting a personal best, it was important for her to set a goal and view it as a starting point.

"It is very helpful for me to think, 'Can I get a little bit faster in the next three months?'" Gabe said. "Reframing goals is definitely a challenge. For someone like me, I'm performance related and I want to see how fast I can run. But at the end of the day, it doesn't really matter how fast I run it. And sometimes I don't even necessarily care if I get back to racing, but I still want to be the best patient I can be."

Gabe's cancer returned in 2017 in the form of metastases on her liver. Despite this, she continued training to find out what was possible despite her diagnosis and to serve as an example to other cancer survivors. "Running is not about my cancer prognosis anymore. It's not about trying to make the Olympics again," she said. "It's about getting some fresh air and clearing my thoughts. Even though I might be slower, or things that used to be easy for me might be a little bit harder, it still improves my day and my overall mindset so much."

Gabe always persevered to live her best life no matter what obstacle stood before her.

"My best advice would just be to not give up on your life and not give up on your health, especially," Gabe told me. "I would encourage people to focus on what you can do. There's always going to be things that cancer takes out of your life or prevents you from doing, which is really frustrating. But the way that I have gotten through ten years of being an intermittent patient is by focusing on what I can do. Sometimes

I'm able to get excited about my performance and still being a fast runner. But on the days that this doesn't motivate me, I'm still motivated by the idea of being the best patient I can be in terms of improving my performance status. Just don't give up. Don't give up on your body."

ACKNOWLEDGMENTS

Kathryn Schmitz

My greatest thanks go to my wife, Sara, for all that she and I have learned, together, since her cancer diagnosis. It was that journey, more than anything else, that inspired this book. I thank Sara, as well as my sons, Mack and Tom, for their patience with the many nights and weekends I have spent writing and editing this work.

Huge thanks to my colleagues who agreed to be interviewed and to share their expertise, as well as the scientists whose work is quoted throughout (regardless of being interviewed). I am humbled to be part of the exercise oncology scientific community and hope that you feel we've represented your work well.

I am grateful to the pioneers of the field of exercise oncology for blazing a trail for so many to follow and the patients who agreed to be studied. We are in your debt.

Finally, thank you to Liz Neporent for her unending friendship and advice, and for introducing me to Gabriel Miller, who has been a joy to work with. Thank you to Michelle Parry for creating the artful, beautiful line drawings contained in these pages. Thank you, Chris Bucci, for taking a chance on me. Finally, I'm grateful to Cara Bedick, for her excellent advice, and for regularly reminding me to have fun along this journey of life.

Gabriel Miller

First and foremost, to be clear: This book would not have been possible without my incredible wife, Kate. To understand her level of support, consider this: I cannot think of a single time in the long effort required to write this book that she questioned a late night or weekend morning spent interviewing, researching, or writing. And this did not simply mean time away from me; while I was off writing, she was solo parenting a six-year old, a three-year old, and a newborn.

Instead, she supported me tirelessly, patiently listening during moments of self-doubt and providing just the right amount of encouragement when an important milestone had been met. To say that I put her on a pedestal vastly underestimates just what I think of her. My only hope is that I can find a way to repay her for this support.

I must also acknowledge my children: to my son Lochlan, who served as a perfect alarm clock for (very) early-morning writing sessions and has shown me what it means to persevere, and to my daughters Adelaide and Camille, who have been genuinely excited that their dad is writing a book. Claudia, Larry, Jeff, and Carol—you have also provided support at key moments.

I owe a deep debt of gratitude to the brave and generous people with cancer who agreed to be interviewed for this book. They shared intimate details so that others could benefit from their experience.

This is also true of the many researchers and oncologists who took the time to answer questions and explain their life's work in lengthy interviews. Their research makes evidence-based books like this possible.

Kathryn Schmitz has been wonderful to work with throughout this entire project. And I need to thank Liz Neporent for her counsel and guidance from the very beginning of this book and Chris Bucci and Cara Bedick for their help and guidance throughout the process.

NOTES

Chapter 1: It Starts with a Phone Call

Page 3: *My most well-known research study:* Kathryn H. Schmitz, et al., "Weight lifting in women with breast-cancer-related lymphedema," *New England Journal of Medicine* 361, no. 7 (2009): 664–73, https://www.nejm.org/doi/10.1056/NEJMoa0810118; Kathryn H. Schmitz, et al., "Weight lifting for women at risk for breast cancer-related lymphedema: a randomized trial," *JAMA* 304, no. 24 (2010): 2699–2705, https://jamanetwork.com/journals/jama/fullarticle/187112.

Page 4: *Thirty-five percent of head and neck cancer patients:* Diane C. Ling, et al., "Incidence of hospitalization in patients with head and neck cancer treated with intensity-modulated radiation therapy," *Head & Neck* 37, no. 12 (2015): 1750–1755, https://onlinelibrary.wiley.com/doi/abs/10.1002/hed.23821.

Page 5: *Women who walked 3 to 5 hours per week:* Michelle D. Holmes, et al., "Physical activity and survival after breast cancer diagnosis," *JAMA* 293, no. 20 (2005): 2479–2486, https://jamanetwork.com/journals/jama/fullarticle/200955.

Page 5: *Dr. Meyerhardt observed a reduction of cancer-specific mortality of over 60 percent:* Jeffrey A. Meyerhardt, et al., "Physical activity and survival after colorectal cancer diagnosis," *Journal of Clinical Oncology* 24, no. 22 (2006): 3527–3534, https://ascopubs.org/doi/10.1200/JCO.2006.06.0855.

Page 5: *A study was published in 1938 with convincing data:* Ivar Sivertsen, "Preliminary report on influence of food and function on incidence of mammary gland tumor in 'A' stock albino mice," *Minnesota Medicine* 21 (1938): 873–875.

Page 5: *In the 1980s, nursing scientists Maryl Winningham and Mary MacVicar:* Maryl L. Winningham and M. G. MacVicar. "The effect of aerobic exercise on patient reports of nausea," *Oncology Nursing Forum* 15, no. 4 (1988): 447–450.

Page 6: *In 1996, two well-known Canadian scientists:* Christine M. Friendenreich and Kerry S. Courneya, "Exercise as rehabilitation for cancer patients," *Clinical Journal of Sport Medicine* 6, no. 4 (1996): 237–244.

Page 6: *At the time, I found twenty-two clinical trials:* Kathryn H. Schmitz, et al., "Controlled physical activity trials in cancer survivors: A systematic review and meta-analysis," *Cancer Epidemiology, Biomarkers & Prevention* 14, no. 7 (2005): 1588–1595.

Page 6: *Five years later, I did the exact same search:* Rebecca M. Speck, et al., "An update of controlled physical activity trials in cancer survivors: A systematic review and meta-analysis," *Journal of Cancer Survivorship* 4, no. 2 (2010): 87–100.

Page 6: *This was followed shortly by similar recommendations:* Cheryl L. Rock, et al., "Nutrition and physical activity guidelines for cancer survivors," *CA: A Cancer Journal for Clinicians* 62, no. 4 (2012): 242–74; Jennifer A. Ligibel and Crystal S. Denlinger, "New NCCN guidelines for survivorship care," *Journal of the National Comprehensive Cancer Network* 11, no. 5 Suppl (2013): 640–644.

Pages 6–7: *The publications from Holmes and Meyerhardt were the first, but dozens:* Anne McTiernan, et al., "Physical activity in cancer prevention and survival: A systematic review," *Medicine & Science in Sports & Exercise* 51, no. 6 (2019): 1252–1261, https://journals.lww.com/acsm-msse/Fulltext/2019/06000/Physical_Activity_in_Cancer_Prevention_and.20.aspx.

Page 7: *And exercise is especially effective in reducing the risk:* Alpa V. Patel, et al., "American College of Sports Medicine Roundtable Report on Physical Activity, Sedentary Behavior, and Cancer Prevention and Control," *Medicine & Science in Sports & Exercise* 51, no. 11 (2019): 2391–2402, https://www.ncbi.nlm.nih.gov/pmc/articles/PMC6814265.

Page 7: *One of these studies took 242 women:* Kerry S. Courneya, et al., "Effects of exercise during adjuvant chemotherapy on breast cancer outcomes," *Medicine & Science in Sports & Exercise* 46, no. 9 (2014): 1744–1751, https://journals.lww.com/acsm-msse/Fulltext/2014/09000/Effects_of_Exercise_during_Adjuvant_Chemotherapy.9.aspx.

Page 8: *And very importantly, there was another group that fared very well:* Kerry S. Courneya, et al., "Effects of supervised exercise on progression-free survival in lymphoma patients: An exploratory follow-up of the HELP Trial," *Cancer Causes & Control* 26, no. 2 (2015): 269–276, https://link.springer.com/article/10.1007/s10552-014-0508-x.

Page 8: *Eight years after surgery:* S. C. Hayes, et al., "Exercise following breast cancer: Exploratory survival analyses of two randomised, controlled trials," *Breast Cancer Research and Treatment* 167, no. 2 (2018): 505–514, https://link.springer.com/article/10.1007%2Fs10549-017-4541-9.

Page 8: *In addition to this type of clinical trial research:* Anne McTiernan, et al., "Physical activity in cancer prevention and survival: A systematic review," *Medicine & Science in Sports & Exercise* 51, no. 6 (2019): 1252–1261, https://journals .lww.com/acsm-msse/Fulltext/2019/06000/Physical_Activity_in_Cancer _Prevention_and.20.aspx.

Page 8: *We were pained to read in the scientific literature:* Kathryn H. Schmitz, et al., "Exercise is medicine in oncology: Engaging clinicians to help patients move through cancer," *CA: A Cancer Journal for Clinicians* 69, no. 6 (2019): 468–484, https://acsjournals.onlinelibrary.wiley.com/doi/full/10.3322/caac.21579.

Page 8: *One recent study of more than 900:* Jennifer A. Ligibel, et al., "Oncologists' attitudes and practice of addressing diet, physical activity, and weight management with patients with cancer: Findings of an ASCO survey of the oncology workforce," *Journal of Oncology Practice* 15, no. 6 (2019): e520–e528, https://ascopubs.org/doi/abs/10.1200/JOP.19.00124.

Page 9: *In one 2019 survey, 95 percent:* A. Smaradottir, et al., "Are we on the same page? Patient and provider perceptions about exercise in cancer care: A focus group study," *Journal of the National Comprehensive Cancer Network* 15, no. 5 (2017): 588–594, https://doi.org/10.6004/jnccn.2017.0061.

Page 12: *A decade later, we can actually prescribe exercise:* Kristin L. Campbell, et al., "Exercise guidelines for cancer survivors: Consensus statement from International Multidisciplinary Roundtable," *Medicine & Science in Sports & Exercise* 51, no. 11 (2019): 2375–2390, https://journals.lww.com/acsm-msse /Fulltext/2019/11000/Exercise_Guidelines_for_Cancer_Survivors_.23.aspx.

Page 12: *And yet, as alluded to earlier, fewer than half of cancer doctors:* Sarah Hardcastle, et al., "Knowledge, attitudes, and practice of oncologists and oncology health care providers in promoting physical activity to cancer survivors: An international survey," *Supportive Care in Cancer* 26, no. 11 (2018): 3711–3719, https://link.springer.com/article/10.1007/s00520-018-4230-1.

Page 12: *The truth, however, is that when faced with a life-changing cancer diagnosis:* Kate Williams, et al., "Health behaviour advice to cancer patients: The perspective of social network members," *British Journal of Cancer* 108, no. 4 (2013): 831–835, https://www.nature.com/articles/bjc201338.

Chapter 2: Now What?

Page 18: *Doing aerobic exercises like walking:* Kerry S. Courneya, et al., "Effects of aerobic and resistance exercise in breast cancer patients receiving adjuvant chemotherapy: A multicenter randomized controlled trial," *Journal of Clinical Oncology* 25, no. 28 (2007): 4396–4404, https://ascopubs.org/doi/10.1200 /JCO.2006.08.2024.

Page 18: *They have found that chemotherapy drugs are distributed more widely:* Jesper Frank Christensen, et al., "Exercise training in cancer control and treatment," *Comprehensive Physiology* 9, no. 1 (2018): 165–205, https://onlinelibrary .wiley.com/doi/abs/10.1002/cphy.c180016.

Page 21: *In one study, they recorded 128 conversations:* Sarguni Singh, et al., "Characterizing the nature of scan results discussions: Insights into why patients misunderstand their prognosis," *Journal of Oncology Practice* 13, no. 3 (2017): e231–e239, https://ascopubs.org/doi/10.1200/JOP.2016.014621.

Page 21: *These are not easy conversations for anyone to have:* Jennifer W. Mack, et al., "Reasons why physicians do not have discussions about poor prognosis, why it matters, and what can be improved," *Journal of Clinical Oncology* 30, no. 22 (2012): 2715–2717, https://ascopubs.org/doi/full/10.1200/JCO.2012.42.4564.

Page 22: *In one analysis that looked at the results of sixty-one clinical trials:* Ben Singh, et al., "A systematic review and meta-analysis of the safety, feasibility, and effect of exercise in women with stage II+ breast cancer," *Archives of Physical Medicine and Rehabilitation* 99, no. 12 (2018): 2621–2636, https://www .archives-pmr.org/article/S0003-9993(18)30280-6/abstract.

Page 22: *A different analysis, this one including the experiences:* Reginald Heywood, et al., "Efficacy of exercise interventions in patients with advanced cancer: A systematic review," *Archives of Physical Medicine and Rehabilitation* 99, no. 12 (2018): 2595–2620, https://www.archives-pmr.org/article/S0003-9993(18)30281-8 /abstract.

Page 24: *Second, there is published evidence that step counts:* Juhi M. Purswani, et al., "Tracking steps in oncology: The time is now," *Cancer Management and Research* 10 (2018): 2439–2447, https://www.dovepress.com/tracking-steps-in -oncology-the-time-is-now-peer-reviewed-article-CMAR.

Chapter 3: The Scientific Evidence

Page 29: *Ten years ago, when the American College of Sports Medicine:* Kathryn H. Schmitz, et al., "American College of Sports Medicine Roundtable on Exercise Guidelines for Cancer Survivors," *Medicine & Science in Sports & Exercise* 42, no. 7 (2010): 1409–1426, https://journals.lww.com/acsm-msse/Fulltext/2010/07000 /American_College_of_Sports_Medicine_Roundtable_on.23.aspx.

Page 30: *Professional distance runner Gabriele "Gabe" Grunewald:* Gabe Grunewald, Bravelikegabe.org, https://bravelikegabe.org/about-gabe. Accessed March 6, 2020.

Page 30: *Renee Seman, a public defender from Long Island:* "She'll run London as her last world major—and it will be her final marathon ever," *Runner's World,*

April 26, 2019, https://www.runnersworld.com/runners-stories/a27275682/renee-seman-running-london-marathon-metastatic-breast-cancer/. Accessed March 6, 2020.

Page 31: *In the 1930s, if you had a heart attack:* Warner M. Mampuya, "Cardiac rehabilitation past, present and future: an overview," *Cardiovascular Diagnosis and Therapy* 2, no. 1 (2012): 38–49, https://cdt.amegroups.com/article/view/108.

Page 31: *In many cases doctors will recommend:* "Heart attack recovery FAQs," The American Heart Association, https://www.heart.org/en/health-topics/heart-attack/life-after-a-heart-attack/heart-attack-recovery-faqs. Updated July 31, 2015. Accessed March 7, 2020.

Page 32: *Following are the areas in which we have the best evidence:* K. L. Campbell, et al., "Exercise guidelines for cancer survivors: Consensus statement from the International Multidisciplinary Roundtable," *Medicine & Science in Sports & Exercise* 51, no. 11 (2019): 2375–2390, https://journals.lww.com/acsm-msse/Fulltext/2019/11000/Exercise_Guidelines_for_Cancer_Survivors_.23.aspx.

Page 33: *It was my own research:* Kathryn H. Schmitz, et al., "Weight lifting in women with breast-cancer-related lymphedema," *New England Journal of Medicine* 361, no. 7 (2009): 664–673, https://www.nejm.org/doi/10.1056/NEJMoa0810118; Kathryn H. Schmitz, et al., "Weight lifting for women at risk for breast cancer-related lymphedema: A randomized trial," *JAMA* 304, no. 24 (2010): 2699–2705, https://jamanetwork.com/journals/jama/fullarticle/187112.

Chapter 4: Finding Motivation

Page 46: *It is often described as the most common, most debilitating:* Victoria Mock, "Fatigue management: Evidence and guidelines for practice," *Cancer* 92, no. 6 (2001): 1699–1707, https://doi.org/10.1002/1097-0142(20010915)92:6+%3C1699::AID-CNCR1500%3E3.0.CO;2-9.

Page 47: *While moving more seems counterproductive at first glance:* NCCN Clinical Practice Guidelines in Oncology, "Cancer-related fatigue," Version 1.2020, 2020, https://www.nccn.org/professionals/physician_gls/pdf/fatigue.pdf. Accessed April 21, 2020.

Page 47: *As just one example, a recent study in Australia:* Dennis R. Taaffe, et al., "Effects of different exercise modalities on fatigue in prostate cancer patients undergoing androgen deprivation therapy: A year-long randomised controlled trial," *European Urology* 72, no. 2 (2017): 293–299, https://www.europeanurology.com/article/S0302-2838(17)30108-2/fulltext.

Page 48: *In another one published in 2017:* Karen M. Mustian, et al., "Comparison of pharmaceutical, psychological, and exercise treatments for cancer-related fatigue: A meta-analysis." *JAMA Oncology* 3, no. 7 (2017): 961–968, https://jamanetwork.com/journals/jamaoncology/fullarticle/2606439.

Page 48: *Knowing that fatigue is the most common side effect:* Ann M. Berger, et al., "Cancer-related fatigue," *Cancer* 118, no. 8 (2012): 2261–2269, https://acsjournals.onlinelibrary.wiley.com/doi/epdf/10.1002/cncr.27475.

Page 53: *When researchers at the Institute of Sport, Exercise and Active Living:* Lindsay G. Smith, et al., "The association between social support and physical activity in older adults: A systematic review," *International Journal of Behavioral Nutrition and Physical Activity* 14, no. 56 (2017), https://ijbnpa.biomedcentral.com/articles/10.1186/s12966-017-0509-8.

Page 53: *Other studies have found that exercising in groups:* Thomas G. Plante, et al., "Does exercising with another enhance the stress-reducing benefits of exercise?" *International Journal of Stress Management* 8, no. 3 (2001): 201–213, https://www.psychologytoday.com/files/attachments/34033/exercise-another.pdf; Dayna M. Yorks, et al., "Effects of group fitness classes on stress and quality of life of medical students," *Journal of the American Osteopathic Association* 117, no. 11 (2017): e17–e25, https://doi.org/10.7556/jaoa.2017.140.

Page 53: *Not surprising, exercising outdoors:* Jo Thompson-Coon, et al., "Does participating in physical activity in outdoor natural environments have a greater effect on physical and mental wellbeing than physical activity indoors? A systematic review," *Environmental Science & Technology* 45, no. 5 (2011): 1761–1772, https://pubs.acs.org/doi/10.1021/es102947t.

Page 53: *Interestingly, the first five minutes of exercising outdoors:* Valerie F. Gladwell, et al., "The great outdoors: How a green exercise environment can benefit all," *Extreme Physiology & Medicine* 2, no. 3 (2013), https://extremephysiolmed.biomedcentral.com/articles/10.1186/2046-7648-2-3.

Page 55: *The following graph, taken from a 1994 publication:* W. L. Haskell, "J.B. Wolffe Memorial Lecture: Health consequences of physical activity: Understanding and challenges regarding dose-response," *Medicine & Science in Sports & Exercise* 26, no. 6 (1994): 649–660, https://journals.lww.com/acsm-msse/Abstract/1994/06000/Health_consequences_of_physical_activity_.1.aspx.

Chapter 5: Prehabilitation (Training Before Treatment)

Page 60: *take a look at the following figure from recent research:* Daniel Santa Mina, et al., "Prehabilitation for radical prostatectomy: A multicentre randomized controlled trial," *Surgical Oncology* 27, no. 2 (2018): 289–298, https://www.sciencedirect.com/science/article/abs/pii/S0960740418300987; Francesco Carli et al. "Promoting a culture of prehabilitation for the surgical cancer patient" *Acta*

Oncologica; 56, no. 2 (2017): 128–133, https://www.tandfonline.com/doi/full/10.1080/0284186X.2016.1266081.

Page 61: *For example, in one study that looked at exercise in more than 49,000 patients:* Daniela Schmid, et al., "Association between physical activity and mortality among breast cancer and colorectal cancer survivors: A systematic review and meta-analysis," *Annals of Oncology* 25, no. 7 (2014): 1293–1311, https://www.annalsofoncology.org/article/S0923-7534(19)36684-0/fulltext.

Page 66: *You could choose to include perceived effort on your log:* Johannes Scherr, et al., "Associations between Borg's rating of perceived exertion and physiological measures of exercise intensity," *European Journal of Applied Physiology* 113, no. 1 (2013): 147–155, https://link.springer.com/article/10.1007/s00421-012-2421-x.

Chapter 6: Surgery

Page 79: *It is a collection of the best and most widely used:* Olle Ljungqvist, et al., "Enhanced recovery after surgery: A review," *JAMA Surgery* 152, no. 3 (2017): 292–298, https://jamanetwork.com/journals/jamasurgery/article-abstract/2595921.

Page 80: *Many studies have shown that moving as soon as possible after surgery:* Xiao Liang, et al., "Enhanced recovery care versus traditional care after laparoscopic liver resections: A randomized controlled trial," *Surgical Endoscopy* 32, no. 6 (2018): 2746–2757, https://link.springer.com/article/10.1007%2Fs00464-017-5973-3.

Page 80: *It is particularly important because the body's tissues decline:* Sue C. Bodine, "Disuse-induced muscle wasting," *International Journal of Biochemistry & Cell Biology* 45, no. 10 (2013): 2200–2208, doi:10.1016/j.biocel.2013.06.011, https://www.ncbi.nlm.nih.gov/pmc/articles/PMC3856924.

Page 80: *As a result, astronauts can lose up to 20 percent of their muscle mass:* National Aeronautics and Space Administration, "Muscle atrophy," https://www.nasa.gov/pdf/64249main_ffs_factsheets_hbp_atrophy.pdf. Accessed August 1, 2020.

Page 80: *Dr. Jessica Scott, a researcher at Memorial Sloan Kettering Cancer Center:* Jessica M. Scott, et al., "Multisystem toxicity in cancer: lessons from NASA's countermeasures program," *Cell* 179, no. 5 (2019): 1003, doi: 10.1016/j.cell.2019.10.024.

Page 97: *Sleep medications that are effective for post-surgery:* Xian Su, et al., "Improve postoperative sleep: What can we do?," *Current Opinion in Anaesthesiology* 31, no. 1 (2018): 83–88, https://www.ncbi.nlm.nih.gov/pmc/articles/PMC5768217.

Chapter 7: Chemo and Other Infusion Therapies

Page 103: *In one study of twenty-seven breast cancer patients:* Amy A. Kirkham, et al., "'Chemotherapy-periodized' exercise to accommodate for cyclical variation in fatigue," *Medicine & Science in Sports & Exercise* 52, no. 2 (2020): 278–286, https://journals.lww.com/acsm-msse/Abstract/2020/02000/_Chemotherapy _periodized__Exercise_to_Accommodate.2.aspx.

Page 104: *The 2019 American College of Sports Medicine Roundtable:* Kristin L. Campbell, et al., "Exercise guidelines for cancer survivors: Consensus statement from the International Multidisciplinary Roundtable," *Medicine & Science in Sports & Exercise* 51, no. 11 (2019): 2375–2390, https://journals.lww.com /acsm-msse/Fulltext/2019/11000/Exercise_Guidelines_for_Cancer _Survivors_.23.aspx.

Page 104: *There is published evidence that cancer patients have a decline in physical function:* Lee W. Jones, et al., "Cardiopulmonary function and age-related decline across the breast cancer survivorship continuum," *Journal of Clinical Oncology* 30, no. 20 (2012): 2530–2537, https://ascopubs.org/doi/10.1200 /JCO.2011.39.9014.

Page 104: *One of my studies shows that exercise can prevent these declines:* Justin C. Brown, et al., "Weight lifting and physical function among survivors of breast cancer: A post hoc analysis of a randomized controlled trial," *Journal of Clinical Oncology* 33, no. 19 (2015): 2184–2189, https://ascopubs.org/doi/10.1200 /JCO.2014.57.7395.

Pages 104–5: *They first looked at 242 women:* Kerry S. Courneya, et al., "Effects of aerobic and resistance exercise in breast cancer patients receiving adjuvant chemotherapy: A multicenter randomized controlled trial," *Journal of Clinical Oncology* 25, no. 28 (2007): 4396–4404, https://ascopubs.org/doi/10.1200 /JCO.2006.08.2024.

Page 105: *As an example, between a quarter and a third of women:* Sara Mijwel, et al., "Effects of exercise on chemotherapy completion and hospitalization rates: The OptiTrain Breast Cancer Trial," *The Oncologist* 25, no. 1 (2020): 23–32, https://doi.org/10.1634/theoncologist.2019-0262.

Page 106: *In their study, 230 men and women with breast or colon cancer:* Hanna van Waart, et al., "Effect of low-intensity physical activity and moderate- to high-intensity physical exercise during adjuvant chemotherapy on physical fitness, fatigue, and chemotherapy completion rates: Results of the PACES randomized clinical trial," *Journal of Clinical Oncology* 33, no. 17 (2015): 1918–1927, https: //ascopubs.org/doi/10.1200/JCO.2014.59.1081.

Chapter 8: Radiation

Page 119: *Yet half of people with cancer require radiation treatments:* Gillian C. Barnett, et al., "Normal tissue reactions to radiotherapy: Towards tailoring treatment dose by genotype," *Nature Reviews Cancer* 9, no. 2 (2009): 134–142, https://www.ncbi.nlm.nih.gov/pmc/articles/PMC2670578.

Page 120: *And in particular, exercise helps with the most widespread problem:* Anand Dhruva, et al., "Trajectories of fatigue in patients with breast cancer before, during, and after radiation therapy," *Cancer Nursing* 33, no. 3 (2010): 201–212, https://www.ncbi.nlm.nih.gov/pmc/articles/PMC2881569/pdf/nihms202882.pdf.

Page 122: *But overall across all of these studies:* Andrea Lipsett, et al., "The impact of exercise during adjuvant radiotherapy for breast cancer on fatigue and quality of life: A systematic review and meta-analysis," *Breast* 32 (2017): 144–155, https://www.thebreastonline.com/article/S0960-9776(17)30021-8.

Page 122: *This same beneficial effect:* Roanne J. Segal, et al., "Randomized controlled trial of resistance or aerobic exercise in men receiving radiation therapy for prostate cancer," *Journal of Clinical Oncology* 27, no. 3 (2009): 344–351, https://ascopubs.org/doi/full/10.1200/jco.2007.15.4963.

Page 123: *More than ten years ago, she presented work:* K. M. Mustian, et al., "A randomized controlled pilot of home-based exercise (HBEX) versus standard care (SC) among breast (BC) and prostate cancer (PC) patients receiving radiation therapy (RTH)," *Journal of Clinical Oncology* 24, no. 18 Suppl (2006): 8504, https://ascopubs.org/doi/abs/10.1200/jco.2006.24.18_suppl.8504.

Page 123: *She later showed that this same at-home exercise program:* K. M. Mustian, et al., "Cytokine-mediated changes associated with improvements in cancer-related fatigue induced by exercise: Results from a randomized pilot study of cancer patients receiving radiotherapy," *Journal of Clinical Oncology* 27, no. 15 Suppl (2009): 9632, https://ascopubs.org/doi/abs/10.1200/jco.2009.27.15_suppl.9632.

Pages 128–29: *Sleep disturbances—whether it be difficulty falling asleep:* Kamala S. Thomas, et al., "Disrupted sleep in breast and prostate cancer patients undergoing radiation therapy: The role of coping processes," *Psycho-oncology* 19, no. 7 (2010): 767–776, https://www.ncbi.nlm.nih.gov/pmc/articles/PMC2922069/pdf/nihms147366.pdf.

Page 130: *In some studies that compare people who get combined chemotherapy:* Stephanie M. de Boer, et al., "Adjuvant chemoradiotherapy versus radiotherapy alone for women with high-risk endometrial cancer (PORTEC-3): Final results of an international, open-label, multicentre, randomised, phase 3 trial," *The Lancet Oncology* 19, no. 3 (2018): 295–309, https://www.thelancet.com/pdfs/journals/lanonc/PIIS1470-2045(18)30079-2.pdf.

Chapter 9: Hormonal Therapies

Page 133: *But many do—in fact, as many of five to eight:* Katherine D. Crew, et al., "Prevalence of joint symptoms in postmenopausal women taking aromatase inhibitors for early-stage breast cancer," *Journal of Clinical Oncology* 25, no. 25 (2007): 3877–3883, https://ascopubs.org/doi/10.1200/JCO.2007.10.7573; Supriya G. Mohile, et al., "Management of complications of androgen deprivation therapy in the older man," *Critical Reviews in Oncology/Hematology* 70, no. 3 (2009): 235–255, https://www.ncbi.nlm.nih.gov/pmc/articles/PMC3074615.

Page 133: *A lot of these people feel so bad:* Marilyn T. Zivian, et al., "Side effects revisited: Women's experiences with aromatase inhibitors," Breast Cancer Action, June 2008, https://bcaction.org/site-content/uploads/2011/03/AI-Report-June-2008-Final-ONLINE.pdf. Accessed September 5, 2020.

Page 137: *For example, several studies have shown:* Katarzyna Hojan, et al., "Physical activity and body composition, body physique, and quality of life in premenopausal breast cancer patients during endocrine therapy—a feasibility study," *Acta Oncologica* 52, no. 2 (2013): 319–326, https://doi.org/10.3109/0284186X.2012.744468.

Page 137: *Exercise also helps prevent the most common side effect:* Melinda L. Irwin, et al., "Randomized exercise trial of aromatase inhibitor-induced arthralgia in breast cancer survivors," *Journal of Clinical Oncology* 33, no. 10 (2015): 1104–11, https://ascopubs.org/doi/10.1200/JCO.2014.57.1547; Hannah Arem, et al., "Exercise adherence in a randomized trial of exercise on aromatase inhibitor arthralgias in breast cancer survivors: The Hormones and Physical Exercise (HOPE) study," *Journal of Cancer Survivorship* 10, no. 4 (2016): 654–662, doi:10.1007/s11764-015-0511-6.

Page 137: *Exercise improves brain function generally:* Cuicui Li, et al., "Can exercise ameliorate aromatase inhibitor-induced cognitive decline in breast cancer patients?," *Molecular Neurobiology* 53, no. 6 (2016): 4238–4246, https://link.springer.com/article/10.1007/s12035-015-9341-9.

Page 137: *Other studies have shown that exercise has a beneficial effect:* Thais R. S. Paulo, et al., "The impact of an exercise program on quality of life in older breast cancer survivors undergoing aromatase inhibitor therapy: A randomized controlled trial," *Health and Quality of Life Outcomes* 17, no. 17 (2019), https://hqlo.biomedcentral.com/articles/10.1186/s12955-019-1090-4.

Chapter 10: Reconstruction

Page 151: *On a scale of 0 to 100, the average satisfaction score:* Katherine B. Santosa, et al., "Long-term patient-reported outcomes in postmastectomy breast reconstruction," *JAMA Surgery* 153, no. 10 (2018): 891–899, https://jamanetwork .com/journals/jamasurgery/fullarticle/2685263; Colleen M. McCarthy, et al., "Patient satisfaction with postmastectomy breast reconstruction: A comparison of saline and silicone implants," *Cancer* 116, no. 24 (2010): 5584–5591, https: //acsjournals.onlinelibrary.wiley.com/doi/full/10.1002/cncr.25552.

Page 151: *On average, four out of every ten:* Laurie E. Steffen, et al., "Met and unmet expectations for breast reconstruction in early posttreatment breast cancer survivors," *Plastic Surgical Nursing* 37, no. 4 (2017): 146–153, https://www.ncbi .nlm.nih.gov/pmc/articles/PMC5951716/pdf/nihms962887.pdf.

Page 151: *Again looking at breast reconstruction:* Katelyn G. Bennett, et al., "Comparison of 2-year complication rates among common techniques for postmastectomy breast reconstruction," *JAMA Surgery* 153, no. 10 (2018): 901–908, https://jamanetwork.com/journals/jamasurgery/fullarticle/2685264.

Page 151: *As Dr. Andrea Pusic, chief of plastic surgery:* Roni Caryn Rabin, "One in Three Women Undergoing Breast Reconstruction Have Complications," *New York Times,* June 20, 2018, https://www.nytimes.com/2018/06/20/well/one-in -three-women-undergoing-breast-reconstruction-have-complications.html.

Page 153: *Because reconstructive surgery by definition involves repairing damaged tissues:* Susan L. Smith, "Functional morbidity following latissimus dorsi flap breast reconstruction," *Journal of the Advanced Practitioner in Oncology* 5, no. 3 (2014): 181–187, https://www.ncbi.nlm.nih.gov/pmc/articles/PMC4114493.

Page 153: *The good news is that exercise helps restore this physical function:* Margaret L. McNeely, et al., "Exercise interventions for upper-limb dysfunction due to breast cancer treatment," *The Cochrane Database of Systematic Reviews* 6 (2010), https://www.cochranelibrary.com/cdsr/doi/10.1002/14651858.CD005211 .pub2/full.

Page 154: *Range of motion exercises may be even more important:* Sandra C. Hayes, et al., "Upper-body morbidity after breast cancer: incidence and evidence for evaluation, prevention, and management within a prospective surveillance model of care," *Cancer* 118, no. 8 Suppl (2012): 2237–2249, https://acsjournals .onlinelibrary.wiley.com/doi/full/10.1002/cncr.27467.

Page 154: *When you look at the results of these studies collectively:* Laurien M. Buffart, et al., "Effects and moderators of exercise on quality of life and physical function in patients with cancer: An individual patient data meta-analysis of 34 RCTs," *Cancer Treatment Reviews* 52 (2017): 91–104, https://www.cancertreatmentreviews .com/action/showPdf?pii=S0305-7372%2816%2930135-9.

Page 154: *It's hard to prove exactly why this is:* Kerry S. Courneya, "Exercise interventions during cancer treatment: biopsychosocial outcomes," *Exercise and Sport Sciences Reviews* 29, no. 2 (2001): 60–64, https://journals.lww.com/acsm-essr/Fulltext/2001/04000/Exercise_Interventions_During_Cancer_Treatment_.4.aspx.

Chapter 11: Post-Treatment

Page 159: *Fatigue is the main one:* Joachim Weis, "Cancer-related fatigue: Prevalence, assessment and treatment strategies," *Expert Review of Pharmacoeconomics & Outcomes Research* 11, no. 4 (2011): 441–446, https://www.tandfonline.com/doi/full/10.1586/erp.11.44.

Page 161: *In fact, as many as one in three cancer patients:* Emily CP LaVoy, et al., "Exercise, inflammation, and fatigue in cancer survivors," *Exercise Immunology Review* 22 (2016): 82–93, https://www.ncbi.nlm.nih.gov/pmc/articles/PMC4755327.

Page 161: *When researchers collect all of the studies:* Shiraz I. Mishra, et al., "Exercise interventions on health-related quality of life for cancer survivors," *The Cochrane Database of Systematic Reviews* 2012, no. 8 (2012), https://www.ncbi.nlm.nih.gov/pmc/articles/PMC7387117.

Page 161: *This stands in stark contrast to drug treatments:* Ollie Minton, et al., "A systematic review and meta-analysis of the pharmacological treatment of cancer-related fatigue," *Journal of the National Cancer Institute* 100, no. 16 (2008): 1155–1166, https://academic.oup.com/jnci/article/100/16/1155/914259.

Page 161: *Just as one example, when researchers looked at more than 12,000 survivors:* Ezzeldin M. Ibrahim, et al., "Physical activity and survival after breast cancer diagnosis: Meta-analysis of published studies," *Medical Oncology* 28, no. 3 (2011): 753–765, https://link.springer.com/article/10.1007/s12032-010-9536-x.

Page 162: *Cancer survivors of all types studied who exercise:* Christine M. Friedenreich, et al., "Physical activity and mortality in cancer survivors: A systematic review and meta-analysis," *JNCI Cancer Spectrum* 4, no. 1 (2019), https://www.ncbi.nlm.nih.gov/pmc/articles/PMC7050161.

Page 162: *When researchers from the American Cancer Society:* Peter T. Campbell, et al., "Associations of recreational physical activity and leisure time spent sitting with colorectal cancer survival," *Journal of Clinical Oncology* 31, no. 7 (2013): 876–85, https://ascopubs.org/doi/10.1200/JCO.2012.45.9735.

Page 162: *Other studies have shown that being sedentary:* A. Ariza-García, et al., "Influence of physical inactivity in psychophysiological state of breast cancer survivors," *European Journal of Cancer Care* 22, no. 6 (2013): 738–745, https://onlinelibrary.wiley.com/doi/abs/10.1111/ecc.12101.

Page 162: *In this study, women with breast cancer who exercised:* Melinda L. Irwin, et al., "Physical activity and survival in postmenopausal women with breast cancer: Results from the Women's Health Initiative," *Cancer Prevention Research* 4, no. 4 (2011): 522–529, https://www.ncbi.nlm.nih.gov/pmc/articles/PMC3123895.

Chapter 12: Survivorship

Page 175: *Two out of every three cancer patients:* American Cancer Society, "Cancer Treatment & Survivorship Facts & Figures 2019–2021," American Cancer Society, 2019, https://www.cancer.org/content/dam/cancer-org/research/cancer -facts-and-statistics/cancer-treatment-and-survivorship-facts-and-figures /cancer-treatment-and-survivorship-facts-and-figures-2019-2021.pdf.

Page 175: *In fact, many people with some of the most common cancers:* N. G. Zaorsky, et al., "Causes of death among cancer patients," *Annals of Oncology* 28, no. 2 (2017): 400–407, https://www.ncbi.nlm.nih.gov/pmc/articles /PMC5834100/#.

Page 181: *In these women, regular physical activity:* Rowan T. Chlebowski, "Nutrition and physical activity influence on breast cancer incidence and outcome," *Breast* 22, Suppl 2 (2013): S30–37, https://www.thebreastonline.com/article /S0960-9776(13)00141-0/fulltext.

Page 181: *In one recent analysis that collected data from sixty-seven previous studies:* Julia Hamer, et al., "Lifestyle modifications for patients with breast cancer to improve prognosis and optimize overall health," *CMAJ* 189, no. 7 (2017): E268–E274, https://www.cmaj.ca/content/189/7/E268.

Page 181: *In another, walking for at least 1 hour a week:* Michelle D. Holmes, et al., "Physical activity and survival after breast cancer diagnosis," *JAMA* 293, no. 20 (2005): 2479–86, https://jamanetwork.com/journals/jama/fullarticle/200955.

Page 182: *There is emerging evidence that exercise might have a positive effect on sexual activity:* Prue Cormie, et al., "Exercise therapy for sexual dysfunction after prostate cancer," *Nature Reviews Urology* 10, no. 12 (2013): 731–736, https: //www.nature.com/articles/nrurol.2013.206.

Chapter 13: Sleep

Page 189: *If you are reading this book because of a recent cancer diagnosis:* Josée Savard, et al., "Cancer treatments and their side effects are associated with aggravation of insomnia: Results of a longitudinal study," *Cancer* 121, no. 10 (2015): 1703–1711, https://acsjournals.onlinelibrary.wiley.com/doi/full/10.1002 /cncr.29244.

Page 190: *At the time of a cancer diagnosis:* Josée Savard, et al., "Cancer treatments and their side effects are associated with aggravation of insomnia: Results

of a longitudinal study," *Cancer* 121, no. 10 (2015): 1703–1711, https://acsjournals
.onlinelibrary.wiley.com/doi/full/10.1002/cncr.29244.

Page 191: *For example, we have strong research showing that with each successive
round of chemotherapy:* Josée Savard, et al., "Breast cancer patients have progressively impaired sleep-wake activity rhythms during chemotherapy," *Sleep* 32, no. 9
(2009): 1155–1160, https://academic.oup.com/sleep/article/32/9/1155/2454469.

Page 191: *When researchers attach Fitbit-like devices to cancer patients:* Heather
S. L. Jim, et al., "Fatigue, depression, sleep, and activity during chemotherapy:
Daily and intraday variation and relationships among symptom changes,"
Annals of Behavioral Medicine 42, no. 3 (2011): 321–333, https://www.ncbi.nlm
.nih.gov/pmc/articles/PMC3432914.

Page 191: *More routinely, people on steroids simply feel very awake:* H. L. Fehm, et
al., "Influences of corticosteroids, dexamethasone and hydrocortisone on sleep
in humans," *Neuropsychobiology* 16, no. 4 (1986): 198–204, https://www.karger
.com/Article/Abstract/118326.

Page 192: *Insomnia is linked to the forgetfulness and difficulty concentrating:*
Kevin T. Liou, et al., "The relationship between insomnia and cognitive impair-
ment in breast cancer survivors," *JNCI Cancer Spectrum* 3, no. 3 (2019), https:
//www.ncbi.nlm.nih.gov/pmc/articles/PMC6640530.

Page 192: *There is even some evidence to suggest that insomnia increases the
risk:* Pasquale F. Innominato, et al., "Subjective sleep and overall survival in
chemotherapy-naïve patients with metastatic colorectal cancer," *Sleep Medicine* 16,
no. 3 (2015): 391–398, https://www.sciencedirect.com/science/article/abs/pii
/S1389945715000556?via%3Dihub.

Page 193: *Again, these results are as good as medications:* Gregg D. Jacobs, et al.,
"Cognitive behavior therapy and pharmacotherapy for insomnia: A randomized
controlled trial and direct comparison," *Archives of Internal Medicine* 164, no.
17 (2004): 1888–1896, https://jamanetwork.com/journals/jamainternalmedicine
/fullarticle/217394.

Page 197: *There are also many studies demonstrating that regular exercise:*
George A. Kelley, et al., "Exercise and sleep: A systematic review of previous
meta-analyses," *Journal of Evidence-Based Medicine* 10, no. 1 (2017): 26–36,
https://www.ncbi.nlm.nih.gov/pmc/articles/PMC5527334.

Page 197: *Another caveat is that while exercise supports good sleep:* Joanie
Mercier, et al., "A non-inferiority randomized controlled trial comparing a home-
based aerobic exercise program to a self-administered cognitive-behavioral therapy for insomnia in cancer patients," *Sleep* 41, no. 10 (2018), https://academic
.oup.com/sleep/article/41/10/zsy149/5059683.

Chapter 14: Nutrition

Page 200: *There is scientific evidence, for example, that maintaining good nutrition:* Christopher G. Lis, et al., "Role of nutritional status in predicting quality of life outcomes in cancer—a systematic review of the epidemiological literature," *Nutrition Journal* 11, no. 27.24 (2012), https://www.ncbi.nlm.nih.gov/pmc/articles/PMC3408376.

Page 200: *In fact, anywhere from 30 to 85 percent:* Federico Bozzetti, et al., "The nutritional risk in oncology: A study of 1,453 cancer outpatients," *Supportive Care in Cancer* 20, no. 8 (2012): 1919–1928, https://www.ncbi.nlm.nih.gov/pmc/articles/PMC3390688.

Page 201: *Several of the largest nutritional studies done to date:* J. L. Krok-Schoen, et al., "Low dietary protein intakes and associated dietary patterns and functional limitations in an aging population: A NHANES analysis," *The Journal of Nutrition, Health & Aging* 23, no. 4 (2019): 338–47, https://link.springer.com/article/10.1007/s12603-019-1174-1; Jeannette M. Beasley, et al., "Dietary intakes of women's health initiative long life study participants falls short of the dietary reference intakes," *Journal of the Academy of Nutrition and Dietetics* 120, no. 9 (2020): 1530–1537, https://jandonline.org/article/S2212-2672(20)30445-7/fulltext.

Page 202: *Research done by the National Cancer Institute:* Elaine B. Trujillo, et al., "Inadequate nutrition coverage in outpatient cancer centers: Results of a national survey," *Journal of Oncology 2019* (2019): 7462940, https://www.ncbi.nlm.nih.gov/pmc/articles/PMC6893237.

Page 204: *For example, the ketogenic diet:* Purna Mukherjee, et al., "Therapeutic benefit of combining calorie-restricted ketogenic diet and glutamine targeting in late-stage experimental glioblastoma," *Communications Biology* 2 (2019), https://www.nature.com/articles/s42003-019-0455-x.

Page 205: *As we have alluded to throughout this chapter:* Christine M. Velicer, et al., "Vitamin and mineral supplement use among US adults after cancer diagnosis: A systematic review," *Journal of Clinical Oncology* 26, no. 4 (2008): 665–673, https://ascopubs.org/doi/10.1200/JCO.2007.13.5905.

Page 205: *Despite how common supplement use is among people with cancer:* Christine M. Velicer, et al., "Vitamin and mineral supplement use among US adults after cancer diagnosis: A systematic review," *Journal of Clinical Oncology* 26, no. 4 (2008): 665–673, https://ascopubs.org/doi/10.1200/JCO.2007.13.5905.

Chapter 15: Caregivers

Page 218: *But there is even some suggestion that if caregivers are depressed:* Kristin Litzelman, "Caregiver well-being and the quality of cancer care,"

Seminars in Oncology Nursing 35, no. 4 (2019): 348–353, https://www.ncbi.nlm.nih.gov/pmc/articles/PMC6728914.

Page 218: *One such report, published in 2013:* Committee on Improving the Quality of Cancer Care: Addressing the Challenges of an Aging Population, Board on Health Care Services, Institute of Medicine; L. Levit, E. Balogh, S. Nass, et al., editors, *Delivering High-Quality Cancer Care: Charting a New Course for a System in Crisis* (Washington, DC: National Academies Press, 2013), https://www.ncbi.nlm.nih.gov/books/NBK202148.

Chapter 16: Athletes

Page 225: *This evidence was highlighted in:* Alpa V. Patel, et al., "American College of Sports Medicine Roundtable Report on Physical Activity, Sedentary Behavior, and Cancer Prevention and Control," *Medicine & Science in Sports & Exercise* 51, no. 11 (2019): 2391–402, https://www.ncbi.nlm.nih.gov/pmc/articles/PMC6814265; Anne McTiernan, et al., "Physical activity in cancer prevention and survival: A systematic review," *Medicine & Science in Sports & Exercise* 51, no. 6 (2019): 1252–1261, https://www.ncbi.nlm.nih.gov/pmc/articles/PMC6527123.

ABOUT THE AUTHORS

KATHRYN SCHMITZ, PhD, MPH, FACSM, is a Distinguished Professor of Public Health Sciences at Penn State University. She is the founding director of the Oncology, Nutrition, and Exercise group at the Penn State Cancer Institute and a past president of the American College of Sports Medicine (ACSM). Dr. Schmitz is the founder of the Moving Through Cancer Initiative of the ACSM, which has a bold goal of making exercise the standard of care in oncology by 2029. She also serves as the Chief Scientific Officer for Maple Tree Cancer Alliance, one of the largest providers of exercise to cancer patients in the United States. Dr. Schmitz has made it her personal mission to use exercise for cancer prevention and recovery, *for all cancers.* Her protocols for exercise in cancer care are used by many major institutions and practitioners. She has presented her research at conferences like the American Society of Clinical Oncology and the American Association for Cancer Research. She has received over $30 million in grant funding from the National Institutes of Health and foundation sources, and published over 260 scientific peer-reviewed papers, including publications in high-tier journals such as the *New England Journal of Medicine* and *JAMA.* Her work has been covered by numerous media outlets, including *Good Morning America,* the *New York Times,* NPR, and the *Wall Street Journal.*

GABRIEL MILLER is a journalist, editor, and author who covers technology, health, and medicine. Though he has written about everything from medical tourism to artificial intelligence for spying, for the last decade he has focused on cancer research. When he's not writing about the latest advances in medicine, he can be found trail running and cross-country skiing in Madison, Wisconsin, where he lives with his daughters, Adelaide and Camille; son, Lochlan; and wife, Kate.

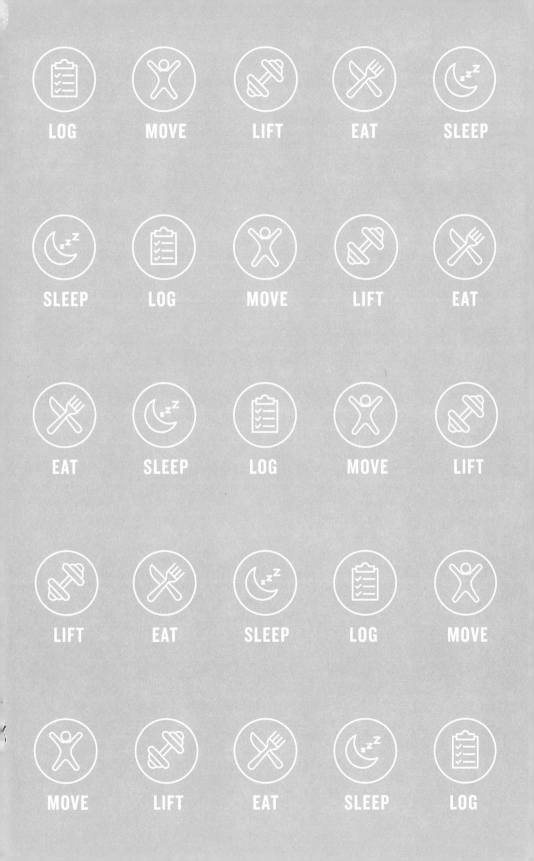

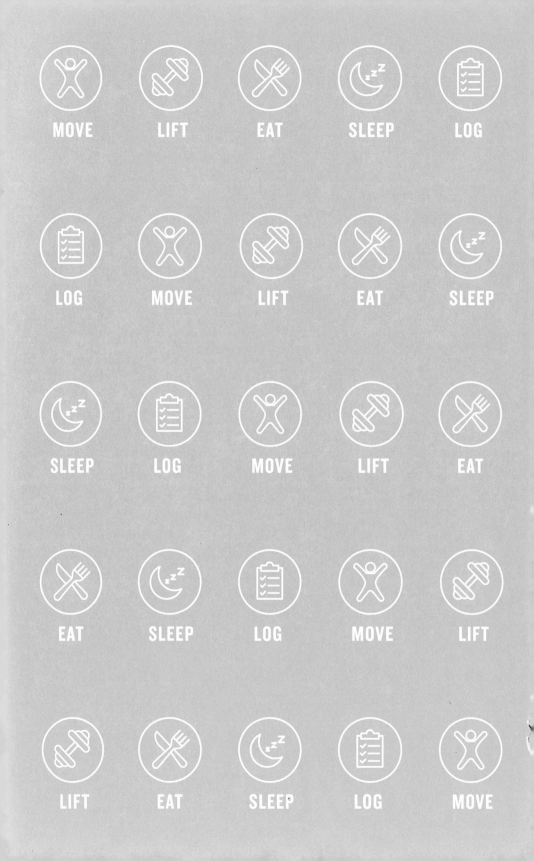